ABC OF PALLIATIVE CARE

ABC OF PALLIATIVE CARE

Edited by

MARIE FALLON

Marie Curie Senior Lecturer in Palliative Medicine
Beatson Oncology Centre, Western Infirmary, Glasgow

and

BILL O'NEILL

Science and Research Advisor
British Medical Association, BMA House, London

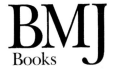

The cover illustration shows a synapse, the junction between two nerve cells.
Other nerve cell bodies are present (branched, with mauve nuclei).
Synapses transmit, electrical signals from one nerve cell to the next. When an
electrical signal reaches a synapse it triggers the release of chemicals called
neurotransmitters (red) from vesicles (pink) in the terminal swelling of the presynaptic
cell. The vesicles burst through the membrane, and neurotransmitters cross a microscopic
gap called the synaptic cleft, and bind to the receptor nerve cell. The Neurotransmitter
changes the permeability of the postsynaptic membrane, causing it to propagate
an electrical impulse.
Reproduced with permission of John Bavosi/The Science Photo Library

© BMJ Books 1998
BMJ Books is an imprint of the BMJ Publishing Group

First published in 1998
Reprinted May 1999
Reprinted 2000
by BMJ Books, BMA House, Tavistock Square, London WC1H 9JR

British Library Cataloguing in Publication Data

A catalogue record for this book is available from the British Library

ISBN 0-7279-0793-X

Typeset by Apek Typesetters Ltd., Nailsea, Bristol
Printed and bound in China

Contents

CONTRIBUTORS

Jim Adam
Consultant Physician in Palliative Medicine and Medical Director,
Hunter's Hill Marie Curie Centre, Glasgow

Julia Addington-Hall
Senior Lecturer in Palliative Care,
King's College School of Medicine and Dentistry,
London

Sarah Allport
Ward Manager
St Oswald's Hospice, Newcastle Upon Tyne

Mary J Baines
Consultant Physician
The Ellenor Foundation, Dartford, Kent

Jennifer Barraclough
Consultant in Psychological Medicine
Sobell House, Churchill Hospital, Oxford

Caroline S Bradbeer
Consultant in Genitourinary Medicine
Guy's and St Thomas's Hospital Trust, London

Eduardo Bruera
Professor of Oncology, University of Alberta
and Director of Palliative Care, Grey Nuns
Hospital, Edmonton, Alberta, Canada

Carol L Davis
Macmillan Senior Lecturer in Palliative Medicine
Countess Mountbatten House, Southampton

Francis G Dunn
Consultant Cardiologist
Stobhill Hospital, Glasgow

Stephen Falk
Consultant in Clinical Oncology
Bristol Oncology Centre, Bristol

Marie Fallon
Marie Curie Senior Lecturer in Palliative Medicine
Beatson Oncology Centre, Western Infirmary, Glasgow

Ann Faulkner
Honorary Professor, the Medical School, Sheffield, and Freelance Author and Lecturer, The Mount, Sheffield

Ann Goldman
CLIC Consultant in Palliative Care
Great Ormond Street Hospital for Children, London

G W Hanks
Macmillan Professor of Palliative Medicine
Department of Palliative Medicine, Bristol Oncology Centre, Bristol

R Johnson
Consultant Anaesthetist
Pain Clinic, Bristol Royal Infirmary, Bristol

Tony O'Brien
Consultant Physician in Palliative Medicine,
Marymount Hospice, Cork, Republic of Ireland

Bill O'Neill
Science and Research Advisor
British Medical Association, BMA House, London

Amanda Ramirez
Professor of Liason Psychiatry, United Medical and Dental Schools of Guy's and St Thomas's Hospitals, London

Claud Regnard
Consultant in Palliative Medicine
St Oswald's Hospice, Newcastle Upon Tyne

Michael Richards
Sainsbury Professor of Palliative Medicine,
United Medical and Dental Schools of Guy's and St Thomas's Hospitals, London

Ann Rodway
General Practitioner, Sevenoaks, Kent

Frances Sheldon
Macmillan Lecturer in Psychosocial Palliative Care, Department of Social Work Studies, University of Southampton, Southampton

Lydia Stephenson
Physiotherapist and Director of Educational Development
St Oswald's Hospice, Newcastle Upon Tyne

J V Sykes
Consultant in Palliative Medicine
The County Hospital, Hereford

John Welsh
Olar Kerr, Professor of Palliative Medicine
Hunter's Hill Marie Curie Centre, Glasgow

Chris Wood
Consultant in Genitourinary Medicine
North Middlesex Hospital, London

Sally Whittet
General Practitioner, Lambeth, London
and Clinical Research Assisitant, Guy's and St
Thomas's Hospital Trust, London

PREFACE

The modern hospice developed with the establishment of St. Christopher's Hospice in London in 1967. The development of services at St Christopher's, both inpatient and home care, signalled a move from previous hospice care based almost entirely on a nursing model with minimal medical support or intervention. It was not until 1987 that palliative medicine was established as an independent specialty. It is hoped that this achievement will be translated into palliative care for all who need it.

Only a small proportion of patients in need of palliative care are cared for in hospices. There is no doubt that the success and relevance of palliative care will be judged not by the number of specialist palliative care units or specialist teams or procedures performed, but by the capacity to influence the care offered to all patients irrespective of diagnosis or place of care.

This ABC is aimed at the primary health care team, hospital doctors, nurses, pharmacists, and students of these disciplines. The principle of palliative care can, and should, be applied to patients at any stage of their illness and not just when they are close to death. A logical systematic and sensitive approach is required to treat the physical and other symptoms suffered by patients. The primary aim of this book is to share the expertise and the evidence, recognising that, as in other areas, the evidence continues to be accumulated to support or refute established practice. We have tried to present the content in an easy to read format. We hope that the book will be a further contribution towards the delivery of palliative care for all and that it will enhance this area of patient care and enable the reader to care for patients with improved knowledge and confidence.

We are grateful to the authors who have shared their expertise and shown patience and forbearance in the production of this book. Without the support of Trish Groves and Greg Cotton and their colleagues at the BMJ Publishing Group the work would never have been finished. We hope that the readers will find that it is of practical use in patient care.

Marie T Fallon
Bill O'Neill

1 Principles of palliative care and pain control

Bill O'Neill, Marie Fallon

Principles of palliative care

'The World Health Organisation defines palliative care as "the active total care of patients whose disease is not responsive to curative treatment. Control of pain, of other symptoms, and of psychological, social and spiritual problems, is paramount. The goal of palliative care is achievement of the best quality of life for patients and their families."

Palliative care is necessarily multidisciplinary. It is unrealistic to expect one profession or individual to have the skills to make the necessary assessment, institute the necessary interventions, and provide ongoing monitoring.

Development of palliative care

Modern palliative care originated in the development of St Christopher's Hospice in London in 1967. Recognising the unmet needs of dying patients in hospital, Dame Cecily Saunders established the hospice and, with others, conceived of a comprehensive approach to dealing with the variety of symptoms and suffering often experienced by patients with progressive debilitating disease. Careful observation of the use and effects of morphine and similar drugs also originated at the hospice.

Traditionally, hospice care was reserved for those with incurable cancer. Increasingly, care is provided for other patients such as those with AIDS and neurological disorders, including motor neurone disease and multiple sclerosis. When palliative medicine was accorded specialist standing in the United Kingdom, in 1987, the agreed definition was "the study and management of patients with active, progressive, far-advanced disease, for whom the prognosis is limited and the focus of care is the quality of life."

In the past hospices provided only inpatient care, and they were isolated from mainstream care. Most units now combine inpatient and home care services, and many independent home care teams also exist, working closely with general practitioners and other workers in primary care. Similarly, many acute hospital and teaching centres now have consultative, hospital based teams.

While hospices will always be needed to care for some patients, the philosophy of care and knowledge gained must be integrated into other specialties. After appropriate assessment, the various methods of symptom control described in this series can be applied at any stage of many illnesses. Symptoms can be relieved while awaiting a response to curative treatment.

Components of palliative care

The essential components of palliative care are effective control of symptoms and effective communication with patients, their families, and others involved in their care. Rehabilitation, with the aim of maximising independence, is also essential to good care. As a disease progresses, continuity of care becomes increasingly important—coordination between services is required, and information must be transferred promptly and efficiently between professionals in the community, in hospitals, and in hospices.

Role of specialists—Most palliative care is provided by general practitioners and by doctors in specialties other than palliative medicine. Specialists in palliative medicine aim to provide care

---

Palliative care

- Affirms life and regards dying as a normal process
- Neither hastens nor postpones death
- Provides relief from pain and other distressing symptoms
- Integrates the psychological and spiritual aspects of care
- Offers a support system to help patients live as actively as possible until death
- Offers a support system to help patients' families cope during the patient's illness and in their own bereavement

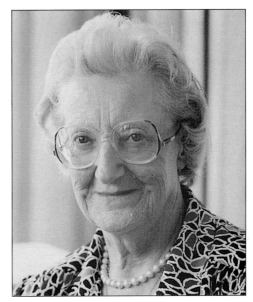

Figure 1.1 Dame Cecily Saunders, founder of St Christopher's Hospice. (Reproduced with permission)

Palliative care services in United Kingdom and Republic of Ireland★

Service	No of units
Inpatient units	223
Beds	3253
Day care centres	234
Home care teams	408
Hospital support teams	139
Hospital support nurses	176

Data from St Christopher's Hospice Information Service

Essential components of palliative care

- Symptom control
- Effective communication
- Rehabilitation
- Continuity of care
- Terminal care
- Support in bereavement
- Education
- Research

for those who need inpatient care or with difficult symptoms, undergraduate and postgraduate education, and research. Education is the key to palliative care for all, and, without research, advances in the science of symptom control and quality of care will stagnate.

Funding—The funding of palliative care services differs from that of the rest of the health service. Only about a fifth of inpatient units in the United Kingdom are funded exclusively by the NHS. Most are funded by the voluntary sector with some financial support from the health service. Although there is a growing partnership between the government and the voluntary hospice sector, voluntary hospices still rely greatly on the goodwill and fundraising initiatives of local communities.

Allocating resources to palliative care

Traditionally, in cancer care, resources were allocated to palliative care only after aggressive attempts to halt the cancer had failed. Palliative care is an integral part of the care of all patients: it does not equate with care at the end of life.

Worldwide, most cancer patients have no hope of cure, and this is particularly true of developing countries, many of which have no screening services for cancer, very limited access to diagnostic facilities, and few specialist cancer doctors. Because of this, the WHO has suggested that, in the developing world, a greater proportion of resources for cancer care should be allocated to palliative care.

While there are serious shortages of essential drugs for pain control, political and cultural attitudes against the use of opioids are major factors in poor control of symptoms worldwide. This highlights the need for national, economic, and political policies on cancer and palliative care.

Principles of managing cancer pain

For most patients, physical pain is only one of several symptoms. Relief of pain should therefore be seen as part of a comprehensive pattern of care encompassing the physical, psychological, social, and spiritual aspects of suffering. Physical aspects of pain cannot be treated in isolation from other aspects, nor can patients' anxieties be effectively addressed when patients are suffering physically. The various components must be addressed simultaneously.

The first principle of managing cancer pain is an adequate and full assessment of the cause of the pain, bearing in mind that most patients have more than one pain and different pains have different causes. A comprehensive knowledge of the underlying pathophysiology of pain is essential for effective management. With effective assessment and a systematic approach to the choice of analgesics, over 80% of cancer pain can be controlled with the use of inexpensive drugs that can be self administered by mouth at regular intervals. Consideration must always be given to treating the underlying cause of the pain by means of surgery, radiotherapy, chemotherapy, or other appropriate measures.

Analgesic drugs

Analgesic drugs form the mainstay of managing cancer pain. The choice of drug should be based on the severity of the pain, not the stage of disease. Drugs should be administered in standard doses at regular intervals in a stepwise fashion. If a non-opioid or, in turn, a weak opioid is not sufficient, a strong opioid is used. Either a weak or a strong opioid should be used, not both.

Adjuvant analgesic drugs may be usefully added at any stage. An adjuvant analgesic is a drug whose primary indication is other than pain but which has an analgesic effect

Some of the national charities—in particular, Macmillan Cancer Relief, Marie Curie Cancer Care, and the Sue Ryder Foundation—are major providers of palliative care, while others such as the National Council for Hospice and Specialist Palliative Care Services, Help the Hospices and the Scottish Partnership Agency do much to promote and support the work of hospices

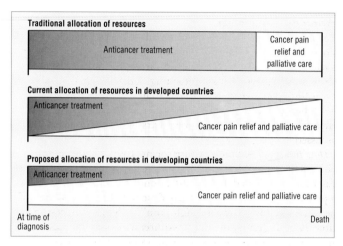

Figure 1.2 Models of allocation of resources for care of cancer patients

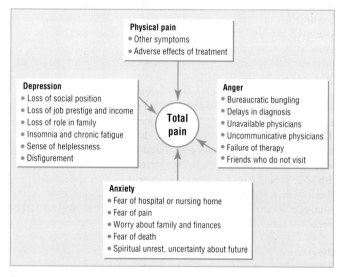

Figure 1.3 Factors affecting patient's perceptions of pain

Analgesic drugs commonly recommended for cancer pain

Mild pain
- Aspirin 600 mg every 4 hours
- Paracetamol 1 g every 4 hours

Moderate pain
- Codeine 60 mg (plus non-opioid drug) every 4 hours
- Dextropropoxyphene 65 mg (plus non-opioid drug) every 4 hours

Severe pain
- Morphine 5-10 mg (starting dose) every 4 hours

in some painful conditions. Examples are corticosteroids, non-steroidal anti-inflammatory drugs, tricyclic antidepressants, anticonvulsants, and some antiarrythmic drugs.

When a non-opioid drug is used together with a weak opioid, many patients find combination formulations more convenient to use. Care must be taken with the dose of each drug in the formulation; some combinations of codeine or dihydrocodeine with aspirin or paracetamol (including co-codamol and co-dydramol) contain subtherapeutic doses of the weak opioid. If these are used and are not effective, more appropriate doses of codeine or dihydrocodeine should be used before moving to strong opioids. The decision to use a strong opioid should be based on severity of pain and not on prognosis.

Strong opioid analgesics

Morphine is the most commonly used strong opioid analgesic. When possible, it should be given by mouth, the dose tailored to each patient, and doses repeated at regular intervals so that the pain is prevented from returning. There is no arbitrary upper limit, but negative attitudes to using morphine still exist; the skilled use of morphine will confer benefit rather than harm, but many patients express fears, which should be discussed.

Dose titration—A quick release formulation of morphine (either elixir or tablet), with a rapid onset and short duration of action, is preferred for dose titration. The simplest method is to prescribe a regular, four hourly dose but allow extra doses of the same size for "breakthrough pain" as often as necessary. After 24 or 48 hours, the daily requirements may be reassessed and the regular dose adjusted as necessary. This process is continued until pain relief is satisfactory. By this method, the many factors that contribute to the variability in dose are taken into account. These include the severity of the pain, the type of pain, the affective component of pain, and variation in pharmacokinetic parameters. The regular dose used may range from 5-10 mg to 2500 mg or more (or the equivalent in controlled release tablets). The dose is titrated against effect, and very few patients need high doses—most require less than 200 mg a day.

Maintenance dose—Patients with advancing disease and increasing pain may require continual adjustment of dose. For many patients, however, there is a period of stability during which the dose required remains unchanged or needs only small adjustments, and this may last for weeks or months or sometimes longer. Once pain is relieved, maintenance will be with a controlled release morphine preparation. Controlled release morphine is available as a once daily preparation that remains effective for 24 hours or a twice daily preparation with effects that last 12 hours.

Alternative routes of administration

The rectal bioavailability of morphine is similar to its oral bioavailability, and it is widely available in suppository form. The rectal route may be appropriate in patients unable to take drugs by mouth, and the same dose as that taken orally should be given four hourly.

For many patients, however, it may be more convenient to convert directly to a subcutaneous infusion of opioid via an infusion device such as a portable, pocket sized, syringe driver. This simple technique allows continuous infusion of opioid analgesics in patients unable to take drugs by mouth. The relative potency of opioids is increased when they are given parenterally: the oral dose of morphine should be divided by two to get the equianalgesic dose of subcutaneous morphine and by three when converting to subcutaneous diamorphine.

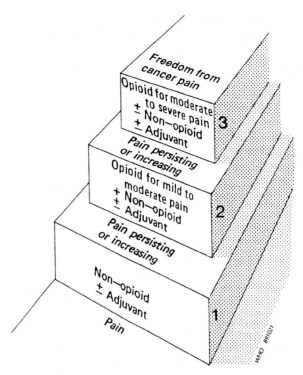

Figure 1.4 WHO's three step ladder to use of analgesic drugs

Opioid alternatives to morphine

Hydromorphone—Has recently become available in Britain. Titration is usually with hydromorphone quick release capsules; when pain is controlled, patients may convert to controlled release preparation. As it is about seven times as potent as morphine, care is needed with patients with no prior exposure to opioids

Fentanyl—Self adhesive patches provide transcutaneous delivery of strong opioid. The patch is changed once every 72 hours. It is used with quick release morphine for breakthrough pain. It is suitable only for patients whose pain is stable because of the time required to titrate the dose upwards. It takes up to 24-48 hours before peak plasma concentrations are achieved

Diamorphine, available only in Britain and Canada, is a semisynthetic derivative and a prodrug of morphine. Use of oral diamorphine is an inefficient way of delivering morphine to the body, but, for parenteral administration, its greater solubility confers an advantage over morphine

Buprenorphine has the advantage of sublingual administration, but it is not recommended except for patients requiring only small doses of opioid

Dextromoramide and *pethidine* are short acting opioids and not appropriate for the management of chronic pain

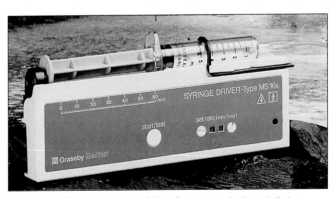

Figure 1.5 Portable syringe driver for automatic drug infusion

3

Rarely, patients may require intravenous administration, and this route may be particularly appropriate for those with an indwelling central line, particularly children.

The indications for administration of strong opioids by intrathecal or epidural routes remain somewhat controversial. There is agreement that patients with pain that is sensitive to opioids who experience intolerable adverse effects with systemic administration may be able to tolerate epidural or intrathecal administration, since much smaller doses of opioid are required to get the same analgesic effect. The more widespread use of these routes is, in general, not justified.

Tolerance and addiction
Tolerance to opioids is rarely seen in the clinical practice of managing cancer pain. Requirements for increasing doses of morphine can usually be explained by progressive disease rather than pharmacological tolerance. Psychological dependence or addiction is not a problem except in patients with pre-existing addiction. If alternative methods of pain control are used (such as nerve blocks) it is usually possible to reduce the dose of the analgesic or even withdraw it without adverse psychological effects.

Opioid toxicity
There is wide variation, both between individuals and over time, in the dose of opioid that is toxic. The ability to tolerate a particular dose depends on the degree of responsiveness of the pain to opioid, prior exposure to opioids, rate of titration of the dose, concomitant medication, and renal function. Toxicity can be a frightening and life threatening experience, but it is usually reversible.

Opioid toxicity may present as subtle agitation, seeing shadows at the periphery of the visual field, vivid dreams, visual and auditory hallucinations, confusion, and myoclonic jerks. Agitated confusion may be interpreted as uncontrolled pain and further opioids given. A vicious cycle then follows, in which the patient is given sedation and may become dehydrated, resulting in the accumulation of opioid metabolites and further toxicity.

Management includes reducing the dose of opioid, ensuring adequate hydration, and treating the agitation with haloperidol (1.5-3 mg orally or subcutaneously, repeated hourly as needed). Subsequent increases in opioid dose may be tolerated.

Opioid responsiveness
Some pains do not respond well to opioids. Although no pain can be assessed as unresponsive to opioids before a careful therapeutic trial of the drug, some pains are more commonly poorly responsive to opioids. These include bone and neuropathic pain. Adjuvant drugs, radiotherapy, and anaesthetic block techniques may be helpful in such cases. Radiotherapy provides effective relief of pain from bone metastases—a single fraction is often sufficient, thus avoiding frequent trips to hospital. Problems with difficult pain will be addressed in the next article in this series.

Common adverse effects of opioids
Sedation—Some sedation is common at the start of treatment, but in most patients it resolves within a few days

Nausea and vomiting—Nausea is common in patients taking oral morphine, vomiting rather less so. These are initial side effects and usually resolve over a few days, but they can easily be controlled—metoclopramide (10 mg every eight hours) or haloperidol (1.5 mg at night or twice daily) is effective for most patients

Constipation develops in almost all patients and should be treated prophylactically with laxatives

Dry mouth is often the most troublesome adverse effect for patients. Patients should be advised on simple measures to combat this, such as frequent sips of cool drinks or sucking boiled sweets, ice cubes, or frozen segments of fruit such as pineapple or melon

---

Common adjuvant analgesics for cancer pain

Drug	Indications
Non-steroidal anti-inflammatory drugs	Bone pain Soft tissue infiltration Hepatomegaly
Corticosteroids	Raised intracranial pressure Soft tissue infiltration Nerve compression Hepatomegaly
Antidepressants Anticonvulsants Antiarrythmics	Nerve compression or infiltration Paraneoplastic neuropathies
Bisphosphonates	Bone pain

The drawings of resource allocation for cancer care, the WHO three step analgesic ladder, and factors affecting perception of pain are redrawn, with permission, from the WHO's *Cancer pain relief and palliative care* (technical report series 804). Geneva: WHO, 1990. The representation of factors affecting patient's perception of pain was based on that first published in Twycross RG, Lack SA, *Therapeutics in Terminal Cancer*, London: Pitman, 1984.

2 Difficult pain problems

J V Sykes, R Johnson, G W Hanks

Roughly 80-90% of pain due to cancer can be relieved relatively simply with oral analgesics and adjuvant drugs in accordance with the World Health Organisation's guidelines. The remaining 10-20% can be difficult to treat.

The terminology used to describe pains that are not easily controlled with opioid analgesics is confusing. It is rarely the case that pain can be described as non-responsive or resistant to opioid analgesics because this implies an all or nothing phenomenon. Usually, pain in cancer responds at least partially to opioids, and a preferable term is "opioid-poorly-responsive pain." A pragmatic clinical definition is that such pain is inadequately relieved by opioid analgesics given in a dose that causes intolerable adverse effects despite optimal measures to control them. The most common example is neuropathic pain.

Neuropathic pain

Neuropathic pain arises from damaged nervous tissue, whereas nociceptive pain results from actual or potential tissue damage. Neuropathic pain may be produced by a tumour infiltrating or compressing nervous tissue, either centrally or peripherally, and may also be caused by surgery, radiotherapy, chemotherapy, or viral infection. Patients may describe the pain as burning, stabbing, stinging, or aching. It may be felt superficially or deeply and be constant or intermittent. It may be spontaneous or precipitated by various stimuli, some of which are not normally painful (allodynia), such as a light touch or cold.

Treatment
Drugs
For most patients a trial of opioids is worth while, usually in conjunction with an adjuvant analgesic. Adjuvant analgesics are drugs with a primary indication other than pain but which are analgesic in some painful conditions.

Non-drug methods
These are used in conjunction with drug treatment, but not all patients find them helpful. Most rely on counterirritation and range from systematic rubbing of the affected part, through application of heat, cold, or chemicals, to acupuncture or transcutaneous electrical nerve stimulation.

Transcutaneous electrical nerve stimulation (TENS) uses surface electrodes connected to a small portable battery to stimulate large diameter nerves in the skin and subcutaneous tissues. Success depends on correct positioning of the electrodes and optimal adjustment of the electrical output, and these differ from person to person. It is relatively free of side effects, but it is difficult to predict which patients will benefit and efficacy often declines over a few weeks.

Acupuncture may be a useful alternative for some patients but depends on local availability of a skilled practitioner.

Physiotherapy may relieve, or prevent the occurrence of, the musculoskeletal problems that can accompany neuropathic pain.

Occupational therapy may teach patients how to regain function without provoking painful episodes.

Useful adjuvant analgesics for neuropathic pain

Our practice is to start with amitriptyline and add an anticonvulsant if the symptoms are not relieved or to substitute an anticonvulsant if the tricyclic is poorly tolerated. If pain is still uncontrolled at this stage, referral for a specialist palliative care opinion or to a pain clinic is advisable

Tricyclic antidepressants—The analgesic effect of tricyclics is independent of any antidepressant effect. Mixed reuptake inhibitors such as amitriptyline seem to be more effective analgesics than the selective serotonin reuptake inhibitors. The starting dose should be low (such as amitriptyline 10-25 mg at night) and then titrated upwards on a weekly basis until pain control improves or side effects become intolerable. An analgesic response has been found with amitriptyline within the range 25-75 mg, but, as the dose increases, so does the frequency of unwanted effects (the evidence of analgesic activity is much less strong for drugs other than amitriptyline)

Anticonvulsants—Doses should start low and be titrated upwards. Sodium valproate (200 mg twice daily, up to 1600 mg a day) is often better tolerated than carbamazepine (200 mg at night, up to 400 mg twice daily)

Antiarrhythmic drugs—These are reserved as second or third line drugs, when treatment with antidepressant or anticonvulsant, or both, has failed. Mexiletine (50-200 mg thrice daily) is usually the first choice in this class

Corticosteroids (for example, dexamethasone 8 mg daily) may be used to reduce inflammation and oedema around a tumour if these are causing nerve compression

---

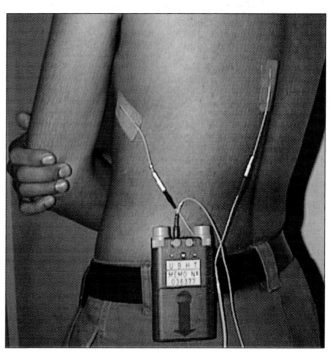

Figure 2.1   Transcutaneous electrical nerve stimulation for control of neuropathic pain poorly responsive to opioids

Incident pain

Incident pain is transient pain precipitated by a voluntary action, such as weight bearing or movement in patients with pain due to bony metastases. It often occurs against a background of adequately controlled baseline pain. An increase in the regular dose of opioid to cover incident pain increases side effects, particularly sedation, when patients are at rest and thus free of pain.

Treatment

Incident pain can severely impair patients' functional ability. Management relies on thorough assessment, treatment of the underlying cause if possible (such as radiotherapy for bone metastases), and optimisation of the analgesic regimen with opioids and appropriate adjuvants by means of "breakthrough doses" in anticipation of pain. For some patients with incident pain, spinal administration of an opioid combined with a local anaesthetic may be worth while, particularly when other treatment options are limited (see below).

Physiotherapy and occupational therapy—Specific rehabilitation in terms of appropriate levels of mobilisation, maintenance of muscle tone and function, ergonomic advice and relevant aids, and necessary changes in lifestyle complement drug treatment and contribute to coping with what may initially seem to be intractable problems.

Surgery—Spinal stabilisation can effectively relieve pain from spinal instability caused by vertebral destruction in a fit patient with a reasonable prognosis (life expectancy of at least three months). Internal stabilisation of a long bone or replacement of a joint may produce considerable benefits even for patients with advanced disease.

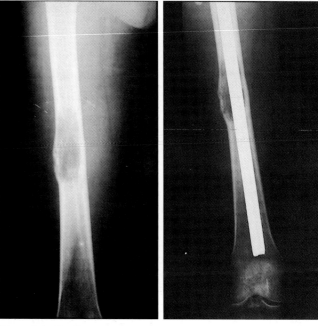

Figure 2.2 Radiographs showing lystic lesion in femur (left) and internal stabilisation of bone (right)

Visceral pain

Visceral pain is often poorly localised and difficult to describe, especially in the early stages, which can make diagnosis of the underlying cause difficult. Localisation often occurs only when disease extends to a somatically innervated structure such as the parietal peritoneum. Abdominal visceral pain is often associated with other unpleasant sensations such as bloating and nausea. Patients may find it difficult to describe the different sensations contributing to their discomfort. There are, however, classic sites of localisation for some organs—such as epigastric pain due to peptic ulcer. Referral of pain to other sites occurs, such as the shoulder tip with diaphragmatic disease or inflammation.

Treatment

As with other types of pain, visceral pain is initially managed with analgesic drugs. However, invasive techniques may be indicated at an early stage. Coeliac plexus block should be considered along with analgesia in patients with pain from carcinoma of the pancreas, not as a last resort. Other upper abdominal malignancies such as carcinoma of the stomach may also benefit from this approach. Visceral pain is nociceptive pain and should respond to conventional analgesics. However, initial good control may be lost as the disease progresses, and a multimodal approach to treatment with drugs and non-drug measures from the outset will produce the best results.

Pelvic tumours may be complicated by bladder and rectal tenesmus, constant severe central perineal pain, and, occasionally, a severe episodic rectal spasm like proctalgia fugax. These pains tend to respond poorly to opioid analgesics, and various other drugs (smooth muscle relaxants, sedative drugs, and anticholinergic drugs) have been advocated. Pharmacological means rarely provide good pain control.

Common causes of visceral pain in cancer patients

- Tumour growth within an enclosed space causing capsular stretch (for example, liver metastases)
- Tumour invasion of parietal (and therefore innervated) surfaces
- Distension and associated muscle spasm provoked by partial or complete blockage of bowel, duct, ureter, or bladder by tumour
- Local inflammation, causing release of pain-producing substances
- Perforation of a viscus
- Occasionally, release of pancreatic enzymes

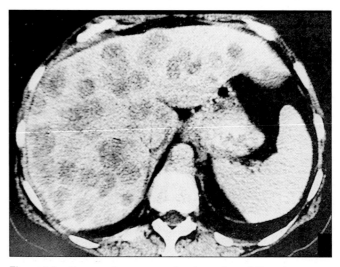

Figure 2.3 Computed tomogram showing enlarged liver due to metastatic spread of cancer

Anaesthetic techniques

In a minority of patients, carefully managed drug treatment, with or without palliative radiation or chemotherapy, fails to provide acceptable pain relief or does so only at the cost of intolerable side effects. In these patients anaesthetic techniques may be indicated.

Spinal administration of drugs

It is now common practice to deliver drugs directly to the central nervous system via fine catheters placed within the epidural space or within the cerebrospinal fluid in the subarachnoid space. Placement is not usually difficult and may be performed under local anaesthesia. Catheters may be tunnelled subcutaneously to exit under the skin at an accessible site. They are attached to a bacterial filter for intermittent or continuous drug administration or, alternatively, may be connected to a subcutaneously implanted reservoir or pump delivery system, which can function for weeks or months.

Drugs—The most commonly used drugs are opioids. Diamorphine has appropriate physical and chemical characteristics to provide good pain relief, and it causes an acceptably low degree of respiratory depression after spread within the cerebrospinal fluid. Other drugs such as dilute anaesthetic solutions and clonidine may be used alone or in combination with opioids to enhance pain control. The 24 hour epidural dose of opioid may be 20-25% of the 24 hour oral dose, and the 24 hour dose to the subarachnoid space is only about 10%. Drugs administered epidurally have to traverse the dura mater to gain access to the spinal cord, and substantial quantities of drug are absorbed systemically both before and during diffusion.

Complications—Infection and mechanical failure of the drug delivery system are not uncommon. Catheters may migrate out of the subarachnoid or epidural space. Implanted reservoirs or pumps occasionally become disconnected from the catheter.

Destruction of nerve tissue

Invasive neurolytic procedures have declined in use because of improved pharmacological management and the relative incidence of adverse effects. However, destructive techniques may provide excellent relief in selected patients.

Coeliac plexus block—The splanchnic innervation of the upper abdominal viscera, notably the pancreas, includes the coeliac plexus. Placement of needles percutaneously, guided by *x* ray or computed tomographic image, permits injection of alcohol or phenol into the nerve plexus. Pain relief may be dramatic and last several months. Early adverse effects are postural hypotension, disturbance of sphincter control, and diarrhoea. Paralysis is an uncommon complication and is most commonly due to damaged arterial blood supply to the spinal cord. Sexual dysfunction is more common.

Subarachnoid neurolysis—Chemicals placed on nerve roots at the level of the dermatomal innervation of somatic pain alter nerve function irreversibly. One example is a neurolytic saddle block in patients with perineal pain due to pelvic malignancy.

Cordotomy lesions are created in the anterolateral tracts of the spinal cord on the opposite side to the pain. Lesions are produced surgically (open cordotomy), or percutaneously by radiofrequency probe passed into the cord guided by *x* ray image. Cordotomy is considered appropriate only for unilateral somatic pain below the fifth cervical dermatome and when life expectancy is less than nine months. Sensory change is an invariable accompaniment, and motor weakness and sphincter disturbances are common. When the operation is provided after proper selection, pain relief may be good for several months.

> Acknowledging that there are situations where adequate pain control may be difficult to achieve is important. A multidisciplinary approach and referral to the appropriate specialist at an early stage can greatly improve the chances of good palliation in these patients

> Spinal opioids are indicated in patients with opioid responsive pain who, when the drug is taken by systemic routes, have intolerable adverse effects at the dose needed for adequate analgesia. The addition of a local anaesthetic may be particularly useful in managing movement related, incident pain

Further reading

Hanks GW, Portenoy RK, MacDonald N, Forbes K. Difficult pain problems. In: Doyle D, Hanks GW, MacDonald N, eds. *Oxford textbook of palliative medicine*. 2nd ed. Oxford: Oxford University Press, 1997

Gybels JM, Sweet WH. *Neurosurgical treatment of persistent pain*. Basle: Karger, 1989

Preconditions for use of neurolytic techniques

- Failure of primary pain management
- Accurate diagnosis of cause of pain
- A condition that responds to neurodestructive techniques
- A risk benefit ratio acceptable to patient, relatives, and clinicians
- Availability of facilities and skills
- Where appropriate, local anaesthetic blocks should be performed before destructive techniques

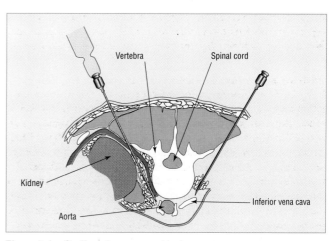

Figure 2.4   Coeliac plexus nerve block

The computed tomogram of an enlarged liver is reproduced with permission of Times Mirror International Publishing.

3 Breathlessness, cough, and other respiratory problems

Carol L Davis

Respiratory problems are common in patients with advanced incurable disease. This article describes palliation of adult patients with malignant disease, but the principles can be applied to many types of non-malignant disease.

A detailed history, examination, and appropriate investigations are needed to establish the most likely cause of any symptom. The history should cover factors that influence the severity of the symptom, including pre-existing diseases (such as chronic obstructive pulmonary disease, which is relatively common in patients with lung cancer), exacerbating factors (such as anaemia, ascites, or profound anxiety), and additional factors (such as pulmonary embolism, infection, or left ventricular failure). All of these will influence management.

Breathlessness

Breathlessness has non-physical as well as physical aspects and, like pain, can be defined by what a patient says it is. It is an unpleasant sensation of being unable to breathe easily. It is relatively common during the terminal stages of cancer: in one survey 70% of 1700 patients with cancer suffered breathlessness during their last six weeks of life. It is a particularly distressing and frightening symptom, not only for patients but also for carers. Activity, levels of anxiety, speed of onset, and previous experience may influence patients' perception of breathlessness and its severity.

While there is often an obvious cause (such as pleural effusion or extrinsic bronchial compression), in some patients no cause is found despite thorough assessment. Little is known about the effects of cachexia on respiratory muscle function, and hyperventilation may account for breathlessness in some cases.

Management

Management of a breathless patient should be individualised, but some general principles apply in all cases. Many members of an interdisciplinary team can contribute. As well as nursing and medical input, physiotherapy is often helpful, particularly for advice on positioning patients in bed, percussion, huffing, control of hyperventilation, and relaxation methods. Practical aids for daily activities are essential.

In selected patients specific treatment such as anticancer therapy can improve symptom control and quality of life. The appropriateness of various strategies varies with time, but, for many patients, the disadvantages of travelling to a distant or regional centre may be justified when weighed against symptomatic relief from radiotherapy, laser therapy, or stenting of an endobronchial tumour. Surgical pleurodesis with insufflated talc should be considered early rather than after repeated pleural aspirations.

Oxygen

Oxygen is usually seen as a non-specific treatment for breathlessness. Patients can become highly dependent on oxygen therapy, and many see it as their lifeline. In patients with chronic lung and heart disease, however, there is good evidence that oxygen therapy is only of benefit in specific situations such as hypoxia or pulmonary hypertension.

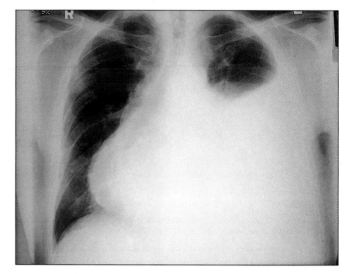

Figure 3.1   Radiograph of patient with malignant pericardial effusion and secondary pleural effusion causing breathlessness

---

General principles of managing breathlessness

- Reassurance to patient, family, non-professional and professional carers
- Explanation
- Advice on positioning patient in bed
- Stream of air—Such as fan, open window
- Distraction and relaxation technique
- Consider blood transfusion if patient anaemic
- Encourage adaptations in activities of daily living, lifestyle, expectations

---

Therapeutic options for specific situations

Pleural effusion
- Pleural aspiration, with or without pleurodesis
- Pleuroperitoneal shunt

Pericardial effusion
- Aspiration, with or without fenestration

Hypoxia
- Oxygen

Lymphangitis
- High dose corticosteroids

Endobronchial disease
- High dose corticosteroids
- Laser therapy
- Cryotherapy
- Stenting

Randomised controlled trials in breathless patients with malignancy are difficult to conduct, and treatment is often based on observational studies and clinical experience. Further research is needed to identify which patients are most likely to benefit from oxygen.

Meanwhile, the pros and cons of oxygen therapy should be considered on an individual basis. The use of nasal speculae rather than a mask can avoid some of the potential problems. The gas can be humidified, but this is noisy. A 24 hour trial of continuous or intermittent oxygen therapy may be appropriate, and it should be accompanied by some form of subjective assessment by patients, with intermittent oximetry if possible. If such a trial of oxygen is successful and relatively long term use is appropriate and anticipated, then an oxygen concentrator rather than cylinders should be considered for patients at home.

Only a small number of patients should require continuous oxygen. For others, explanation combined with non-specific drug measures, especially anxiolytics, and possibly a bedside or hand held fan can have dramatic effects, sometimes removing the need for oxygen therapy even in patients apparently "glued" to their masks.

Benzodiazepines
Anxiolytics, particularly benzodiazepines, have a place in managing breathlessness even in patients who do not have prominent anxiety or panic attacks. Low doses of benzodiazepines can cause substantial improvement in some patients, and concern about possible respiratory depression is usually unfounded—any such concern should be weighed against the potential benefit of treatment. Benzodiazepines probably relieve breathlessness through anxiolytic and sedative effects and, possibly, muscle relaxation.

The vicious cycle in which anxiety aggravates breathlessness and breathlessness in turn creates further anxiety is experienced to some degree by most breathless patients, regardless of the cause of the symptom. Some patients may experience a severe panic attack and become convinced that they are about to die. Such attacks are more common than is acknowledged. Patients should be advised of measures that they can initiate and which allow them to regain control. These have been summarised as "Stop, purse lips, drop (shoulders), and flop."

Opioids
The relation between opioids and respiration is not simple; if used inappropriately, opioids can induce respiratory depression, which is determined by pathophysiology, prior exposure to opioids, rate and route of dose titration, and coexisting pathology. However, low dose oral opioids can improve breathlessness, sometimes dramatically, although the precise mechanism of action is unknown.

The dose of opioid can be titrated in the same way as when used for pain control, but lower doses and smaller increments should be used. In patients not previously exposed to opioids, as little as 2.5 mg of morphine elixir every 4 hours may be sufficient. If a patient is already receiving controlled release morphine, it is usual to convert to a quick release preparation and allow for a dose increment. For patients unable to swallow, subcutaneous diamorphine can be used. In almost all cases concurrent laxatives should be prescribed.

Trials of nebulised morphine have been conducted in healthy volunteers and in patients with chronic obstructive pulmonary disease and with breathlessness due to malignant disease. The current evidence does not support their use. In any case, bronchospasm, particularly at higher doses, can be a problem, and there is no consensus on the optimal drug, dose, schedule of administration, or method of dose titration.

Pros and cons of oxygen therapy

Potential advantages	Potential disadvantages
• Reverses hypoxia	• Ties patient to oxygen source
• Improved wellbeing in some patients	• Potential loss of respiratory drive
• Placebo effect	• Claustrophobia
Patient	• Difficulty in talking
Relatives	• Distancing
Professionals	• Dry mouth
	• Cost

Choices of anxiolytic drug for treating breathlessness

Lorazepam (0.5-2 mg) can be taken sublingually and is rapidly absorbed with a rapid onset of action and a short half life. It is particularly useful for self administration during an episode of acute breathlessness

Diazepam (starting dose usually 5 mg daily) is preferred if a regular anxiolytic is required. Some patients require much higher doses. With a half life of 30-60 hours, it can be administered as a single bedtime dose, orally or rectally

Midazolam—If parenteral administration is required, midazolam can be given by subcutaneous injection (initially 2.5-5 mg) or by infusion (starting dose 10 mg/24 hours, increasing as necessary), often in combination with low dose diamorphine

Methotrimeprazine, a phenothiazine with profound sedating properties at higher doses (and antiemetic properties), is occasionally used as an alternative to midazolam

---

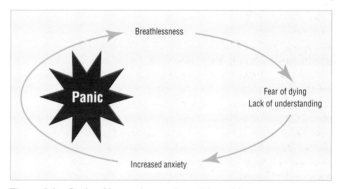

Figure 3.2   Cycle of increasing panic and breathlessness

Advice to patient about "panic attacks"
• Try to stay calm
• Purse your lips
• Relax shoulders, back, neck, and arms
• Concentrate on breathing out slowly (if breathing in seems difficult)

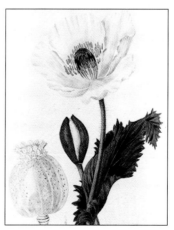

Figure 3.3   The opium poppy, *Papavers somniferum*

Other drugs

Traditionally, other drugs are more commonly administered via nebulisers. If a trial of such a drug is thought appropriate, then nebulised normal saline should be used in the first instance. Inhaled bronchodilators should be reserved for patients with reversible airways obstruction. Other nebulised drugs should be regarded as experimental in this population of patients.

Cough

Cough is a normal but complex physiological mechanism that protects the airways and lungs by removing mucus and foreign matter from the larynx, trachea, and bronchi and is under both voluntary and involuntary control. Pathological cough is common in malignant and non-malignant disease. Cough can be classified in various ways, and several causes may coexist in one patient.

Management

Management should be determined by the type and the cause of the cough as well as the patient's general condition and likely prognosis. When possible, the main aim should be to reverse or ameliorate the cause, combined with appropriate symptomatic measures. Exacerbating factors should be defined, and simple measures such as a change in posture, particularly at night, can be very helpful.

Breathlessness can trigger cough, and vice versa. Persistent cough can also precipitate vomiting, exhaustion, chest or abdominal pain, rib fracture, syncope, and insomnia, and these problems may need to be addressed.

Cough suppressants are usually used to manage dry, but not productive, cough, except in irritant nocturnal cough and cough in dying patients. The most effective antitussive agents are the opioids. Codeine linctus is a mild antitussive while the strong opioids have a more pronounced effect. Methadone linctus can be particularly effective at night, because it has a long half life, but the risk of accumulation exists.

Mucolytic treatments such as simple linctus or nebulised saline may benefit patients with a wet unproductive cough. Use of nebulised saline can result in bronchaspasm and the production of copious liquid sputum, and this makes it unsuitable for those who are unable to expectorate.

Nebulised local anaesthetics can relieve intractable and unproductive cough for which no other treatment has been found. Bronchospasm can occur and not necessarily only with the first dose—nebulised bronchodilators should therefore be available, at least when treatment is initiated. Both lignocaine (up to 5 ml of 2% solution every 6 hours) and bupivacaine (up to 5 ml of 0.25% solution every 8 hours) have been used. The relative efficacy and toxicity of these agents have not been established, and treatment reduces the sensitivity of the gag reflex and causes a transitory hoarse voice. Patients should not eat or drink for an hour after nebulisation.

Antibiotics can be used, even in dying patients, to relieve a productive cough that is causing pain, insomnia, or distress. The decision on whether to treat an infection with antibiotics may raise ethical dilemmas and needs careful consideration and discussion. Appropriate chest physiotherapy should be considered in all patients including those close to death.

Antimuscarinics—In some patients it is more appropriate to reduce salivary secretions. Hyoscine hydrobromide can be given as a subcutaneous injection (0.2-0.4 mg, repeated as necessary) or by subcutaneous infusion over 24 hours (1.2-2.4 mg). It has central side effects, causing sedation and occasionally dysphoria. If these are problematic, glycopyrronium bromide is an alternative option.

Common causes of cough

Non-malignant

Acute infection
- Upper respiratory viral infection
- Bronchopneumonia

Airway disease
- Asthma
- Chronic obstructive pulmonary disease

Irritant
- Foreign body
- Cigarette smoke
- Oesophageal reflux

Cardiovascular causes
- Left ventricular failure

Malignant

Airway obstruction
- Endobronchial disease

Pleural disease
- Pleural effusion
- Mesothelioma

Chronic infection
- Cystic fibrosis
- Bronchiectasis
- Postnasal drip

Parenchymal disease
- Interstitial fibrosis

Recurrent aspiration
- Motor neurone disease
- Multiple sclerosis

Drug induced
- Angiotensin converting enzyme inhibitors
- Inhaled drugs

Interstitial disease
- Lymphangitis
- Multiple pulmonary metastases
- Radiation pneumonitis

Vocal cord palsy
- Hilar tumour or lymphadenopathy

Classification of types of cough

- Productive cough, patient able to cough effectively
- Productive cough, patient not able to cough effectively
- Non-productive cough

Pharmacological agents that inhibit cough

Opioids and opioid derivatives
- Codeine phosphate
- Dextromethorphan
- Pholcodine
- Methadone
- Morphine

Local anaesthetics

Lozenges
- Benzocaine
- Lignocaine
  For laryngeal, pharyngeal, or tracheal irritation

Nebulised
- Lignocaine
- Bupivacaine
  Useful for intractable, unproductive cough (with care)

Corticosteriods
- Prednisolone
- Dexamethasone
  Often used to relieve cough related to endobronchial tumour, lymphangitis, or radiation pneumonitis

Bronchodilators
- Salbutamol
- Ipratropium
  Can relieve cough associated with chronic obstructive pulmonary disease

---

Therapeutic options in managing productive cough

Tenacious sputum
- Steam inhalation
- Nebulised saline
- Simple linctus
- Physiotherapy
- (Cough suppression)

Heart failure
- Diuretics

Purulent sputum
- Antibiotics
- Postural drainage
- Physiotherapy
- Cough suppression

Loose secretions but unable to cough
- Positioning
- Hyoscine hydrobromide
- Glycopyrronium bromide
- Suction

Haemoptysis

In many studies of patients with haemoptysis a definite cause is established in only half of cases. Even in patients with a proved malignancy, haemoptysis can be due to other causes. While lung cancer is the commonest cause of massive haemoptysis (>200 ml/24 hours), non-malignant disorders such as acute bronchitis, bronchiectasis, and pulmonary embolism can cause mild to moderate haemoptysis.

Management

It is important to establish that the blood or blood stained material has come from the chest and not the nose, upper respiratory tract, or gastrointestinal tract. Management depends on the cause and prognosis. Radiotherapy (endobronchial or external beam) and laser therapy are particularly effective in controlling bleeding from endobronchial tumour.

Massive haemoptysis should be regarded as an emergency whether or not resuscitation is appropriate. Patients bleeding as a result of a non-malignant cause such as aspergilloma, lung abscess, or bronchiectasis may warrant active management, but this is rarely the case in patients with haemoptysis and lung malignancy receiving palliative care.

Palliative management should be aimed at reducing awareness and fear. A combination of a parenterally administered strong opioid and a benzodiazepine is usually required. The intravenous route should be used if there is peripheral vascular shutdown. It is often possible to predict the likelihood of a massive bleed and to plan for such a crisis in several ways, including establishing an emergency supply of appropriate drugs in the patient's home. Careful judgment is required in deciding whether to discuss the risk of massive haemoptysis with a patient and relatives.

Therapeutic options for haemoptysis	
Minor bleed	**Major bleed**
Caused by lung tumour	*Resuscitation appropriate*
● Oral haemostatic drug—Such as tranexamic acid or ethamsylate	● Establish intravenous access
	● Transfusion
● Radiotherapy—External beam or endobronchial	● Bronchoscopy and endoscopic measures
● Laser therapy	● Bronchial artery embolisation
	● Open surgery
Caused by pulmonary embolism	*Resuscitation inappropriate*
● Anticoagulation	● Intravenous opioid and benzodiazepine
Any cause	*Both situations*
● Treat coagulation disorder if present	● Nurse patient lying on his or her side, on the side of the tumour
● Cough suppressant	● Mask evidence of bleed—Such as with red or green towels
	● Calm witnesses—Patient, family, staff, other patients

Stridor

A harsh inspiratory wheezing sound results from obstruction of the larynx or major airways. Treatment with corticosteroids (such as dexamethasone 16 mg daily) can provide rapid relief. Explanation should always be given, together with advice about sitting or lying as upright as possible and measures to relieve anxiety. Radiotherapy or endoscopic insertion of a tracheal or bronchial stent should be considered but are not always appropriate. Inhalation of a mixture of helium and oxygen (in a ratio of 4:1) is used in some centres.

Pleural and chest wall pain

Pleural and chest wall pain may exacerbate breathlessness and may be difficult to manage. Analgesics should be prescribed in a step-wise fashion as detailed in the first article in this series. If a patient also has a cough then cough suppression will help. Radiotherapy should be considered if the pain is caused by bone or soft tissue metastases. An intercostal nerve block may alleviate pain from rib metastases or fracture.

Conclusion

Patients and their lay and professional carers need to acknowledge that respiratory problems, particularly breathlessness, can be difficult to palliate. A patient centred, problem orientated approach is required. Professionals from many different specialties and disciplines have a potential role. Few of the management strategies discussed above have been submitted to adequate scientific scrutiny, and there is urgent need for further research.

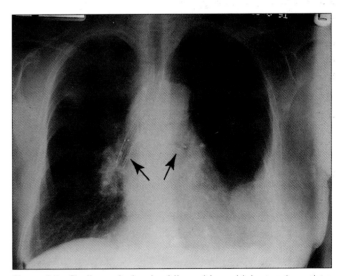

Figure 3.4 Radiograph showing bilateral bronchial stents in patient with obstructive lesion

The picture of the opium poppy is reproduced courtesy of the Royal Botanical Gardens, Kew.

4 Mouth care, skin care, and lymphoedema

Claud Regnard, Sarah Allport, Lydia Stephenson

Mouth care

Patients' oral problems can be kept to a minimum by good hydration, brushing the teeth with a fluoride toothpaste twice daily, and daily observation of the oral mucosa. Oral problems can reduce intake of fluid and food because of pain, altered taste, or disorders of swallowing. The first step is to manage the local problems.

Infection

Candidiasis usually presents as adherent white plaques but can also present as erythema or angular cheilitis. Nystatin suspension is the usual treatment, but in advanced disease ketoconazole 200 mg once daily for 5 days is cost effective and more convenient for patients (hepatic toxicity has not been reported for 5 day courses). Fluconazole 150 mg as a single dose is equally effective but is more expensive. Recurrent candidiasis in patients with AIDS requires prophylactic treatment with fluconazole 50 mg daily.

Oral hygiene is important, especially daily cleaning of dentures. Aphthous ulcers are common and can be helped by topical corticosteroids or tetracycline mouthwash. Severe viral infection (herpes simplex or zoster) will need aciclovir 200 mg every 4 hours for 5 days. Malignant ulcers are often associated with anaerobic bacteria that produce a foul odour; this responds to metronidazole, either as 400-500 mg taken orally or rectally every 12 hours or as a topically applied gel.

Dirty mouth

Loose oral debris can be removed with mouthwashes. Over the years many different mouthwashes have been advocated and then rejected for various reasons. Cider and soda water are more pleasant than most, while cool water is by far the most convenient. Teeth should be brushed at least twice daily with a fluoride toothpaste. Dental caries, if present, should prompt referral to a dentist. A coated tongue can be cleared in days with the proteolytic enzyme annanase, effectively delivered by regular chewing of unsweetened pineapple chunks (annanase remains fully active in tinned fruit).

Dry mouth

Treatable causes include candidiasis, antimuscarinic drugs, anxiety, and dehydration. Helpful local measures include partly frozen drinks, while frequent sips or sprays of plain cold water are as effective as artificial salivas. Applying petroleum jelly to the lips prevents sore cracked lips. Glycerin, which dehydrates the mucosa further, and lemon juice, which rapidly exhausts salivary secretion, should be avoided.

Painful mouth

In patients with head and neck tumours infection can cause sudden and severe pain with little or no signs, but it responds rapidly to systemic flucloxacillin and metronidazole. Pain from bone or nerve damage is treated as described earlier in this series. Persistent mucosal pain is helped by topical measures: some provide local protection, and others produce local anaesthesia. Severe pain due to mucositis occasionally needs systemic analgesics such as opioids, with the dose titrated against the pain.

Risk factors for oral problems

- Debility
- Dry mouth
- Chemotherapy
- Poor oral intake
- Local irradiation
- Dehydration

Key questions for mouth care

- Is infection present?
- Is the mouth dry?
- Is the mouth dirty?
- Is the mouth painful?

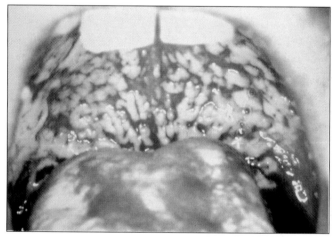

Figure 4.1 Oral candidiasis

Local measures for oral problems

Infected mouth
- Topical corticosteroids—Betamethasone 0.5 mg in 5 ml water as mouthwash or triamcinolone in carmellose paste
- Tetracycline mouthwash, 250 mg every 8 hours (contents of one capsule dissolved in 5 ml water)

Dirty mouth
- Regular brushing with soft toothbrush and toothpaste
- Pineapple chunks
- Cider and soda mouthwash

Dry mouth
- Semifrozen tonic water and gin
- Semifrozen fruit juice
- Frequent sips of cold water or water sprays
- Petroleum jelly rubbed on lips

Painful mouth
- Coating agents—Sucralfate suspension as mouthwash, carmellose paste, carbenoxolone
- Topical anaesthesia—Benzydamine mouthwash, choline salicylate, Mucaine, lozenges containing local anaesthetics

Skin care

Pressure sores

Patients at risk of pressure sores should be monitored regularly with a validated risk assessment score (such as Waterlow) and daily visual inspection of pressure areas. How a patient moves, or is moved by carers, needs to be assessed and monitored. Even with regular turning and careful lifting and positioning, specialist pressure surfaces or mattresses are sometimes needed.

Painful pressure sore—Gel or colloid dressings that keep the area moist reduce pain and can be left in place for several days. Topical application of benzydamine to the edges of the ulcer can also help. Painful changing of dressings can be eased by extra analgesia before each change. Inhaling a mixture of oxygen and nitrous oxide (Entonox) may help, but persistent pain may require oral diclofenac or oral morphine. Severe pain may need a subcutaneous infusion of ketamine (50-200 mg per 24 hours) or spinal analgesia.

Odour—Anaerobic bacteria causing odour can be reduced with systemic metronidazole 400-500 mg taken orally or rectally twice daily. Topical metronidazole gel is an expensive alternative if systemic metronidazole is not tolerated. Perfumes are unhelpful as they soon become associated with the unpleasant odour.

Patient's prognosis—When there is insufficient time to allow healing, care should focus on preventing worsening of pressure sores, comfortable dressings, pain relief, and reducing odour. Solutions that release chlorine, such as Eusol and Milton, seem to delay healing.

Nutrition—Good hydration, high protein and carbohydrate drinks, and vitamin C supplements encourage healing.

Faecal or urinary contamination—No pressure sore is free of bacterial contamination, but diarrhoea or urinary incontinence will make healing more difficult, and this should be addressed separately.

Suitability of dressings—It is important to check that the required dressings can be prescribed (listed in the *Drug Tariff*) and that someone can collect them for the patient. Planning between hospital, hospice, and community is essential and, if necessary, one care team should demonstrate the dressing technique to other teams.

Malignant ulcers

Uncomplicated malignant ulcers, pain relief and wound care are managed in the same way as pressure sores, but many malignant ulcers present special problems requiring additional treatment.

Bleeding ulcer—Radiotherapy should be arranged. While awaiting treatment, or if there is no further scope for treatment, bleeding points or capillary oozing can be successfully managed by topical application of sucralfate. The suspension is placed on a non-adherent dressing and applied firmly to the bleeding area. An alternative is the topical application of tranexamic acid injection solution. The duration of action of topical adrenaline is too short to be useful in bleeding ulcers.

Altered body image—Odour is managed in the same way as with pressure sores, while cosmetic camouflage and filling cavities with cavity foam dressings can restore some symmetry. Both odour and asymmetry can cause social isolation, altered body image, and sexual difficulties with resultant psychosocial difficulties. Empathetic listening is often therapeutic in itself, but anxiety, anger, or depression will need specific support.

Dirty ulcer—If the prognosis allows, debridement can be gently achieved with polysaccharide, hydrocolloid, or hydrogel dressings. Odour is treated in the same way as for pressure sores, but, for extra masking of the odour, cling film (food wrap) can be placed over the outermost dressing.

Risk factors for pressure sores
- Debility
- Dyspnoea
- Incontinence
- Confusion
- Pain
- Paralysis
- Poor nutrition
- Weakness

Likely site of pressure damage
- Shoulder blades
- Elbows
- Spine
- Buttocks
- Knees
- Ankles
- Heels

Key questions in managing pressure sores
- Is the pressure sore painful?
- Is the odour present?
- Will patient's prognosis allow healing?
- Is better nutrition possible?
- Is the ulcer dirty?
- How deep is the ulcer?
- Is faecal or urinary contamination present?
- Are the dressings practical and available?

Dressings for ulcers

Shallow ulcers (<5 mm deep)—Use a moisture retaining dressing such as hydrocolloid wafers or adhesive semipermeable films

Deep ulcers (≥5 mm)—Use a moist cavity dressing to encourage granulation (such as calcium alginate hydrogel or cavity foam dressing)

Heavy exudate—Calcium alginate is preferable

Slough and necrotic tissue—Apply hydrocolloid or hydrogel dressing for a week, then debride gently

---

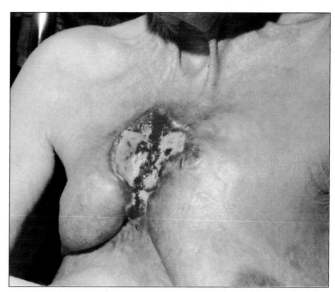

Figure 4.2 Malignant ulcer in 65 year old woman previously treated for breast cancer

Excessive discharge—High absorbency dressings such as calcium alginate take up some discharge, and the surrounding skin will need a barrier ointment. Profuse watery discharge from some ulcers can be greatly reduced by using topical high dose corticosteroids once daily for a week. If the discharge is due to an enterocutaneous fistula, a stoma bag may help if surgical diversion is not possible, but occasionally octreotide (starting dose 150-300 µg per 24 hours) can reduce the volume of the enteral discharge. Bed linen can rapidly become soiled—for patients at home, the community laundry service should be contacted, while the local authority can usually arrange for the safe and discrete collection of linen.

Itch

Skin unusually dry or wet—If the skin is dry avoid heat, hot baths, drying agents such as calamine, and rough clothing. Moisturise the skin regularly with an emollient such as aqueous cream. For wet skin, use barrier cream in skin folds and, after washing, dry the skin without rubbing. Reduce sweating by treating infection or reduce fever by cooling. Night sweats can be difficult to treat: thioridazine (10-30 mg at night), corticosteroids, cimetidine, and non-steroidal anti-inflammatory drugs have shown some success. Dermatitis and atopic eczema usually cause dry skin but can cause wetness if the irritation is acute or has been excoriated. The associated itch can be rapidly eased with topical corticosteroids—the risk of systemic absorption is much less of a problem in advanced disease.

Skin colour change—Consider iron deficiency anaemia and jaundice as causes. Jaundice due to biliary obstruction caused by malignancy can be relieved by stenting, or temporarily eased by high dose dexamethasone. Darkening of the skin may be due to poor venous drainage, ischaemia, or local tumour.

Skin damaged—Consider infection, pressure damage, and skin disorders.

Persistent itch—When itch persists despite local measures (emollients such as aqueous cream, with topical corticosteroids if necessary) systemic drug therapy can be tried: antihistamines, chlorpromazine, cholestyramine, cimetidine, phenobarbitone, and rifampicin help some patients, and, recently, ondansetron has been suggested for itch secondary to cholestatic jaundice. The variety of drugs emphasises the uncertain success of drug treatments and reinforces the importance of local measures.

Lymphoedema

Low protein oedemas (such as those due to heart failure, dependency, or hypoalbuminaemia) are soft and are managed by low compression support, elevation, and treating the underlying cause. Lymphoedema, however, results from reduced lymphatic drainage, which can be caused by lymphatic obstruction due to tumour, infection, or scarring.

Affected tissues are initially soft, and the lymphoedema may reduce or disappear overnight, but within a year or two the tissues become firm with deep folds, a dry roughened skin, and, eventually, hyperkeratosis and recurrent cellulitis. Patients may complain of stiffness or pain from related conditions (such as cellulitis or a heavy limb), but lymphoedema itself is not painful. Lymphoedema alone never causes skin ulceration or nerve damage, and other causes must be sought if these are present.

Infection

Cellulitis is usually due to penicillin sensitive *Streptococcus*, although skin swabs are often unhelpful. The infection often causes only mild erythema and increased warmth, although acute infection can occur. Prompt treatment with penicillin V

Key questions in managing malignant ulcers?

- Is the ulcer bleeding?
- Is the ulcer dirty?
- Is discharge excessive?
- Is ulcer painful or itching?
- Does patient have an altered body image?

Key questions in managing itch

- Is skin drier or wetter than usual?
- Has skin colour changed?
- Is skin abnormal?
- Is itch persisting despite local measures?

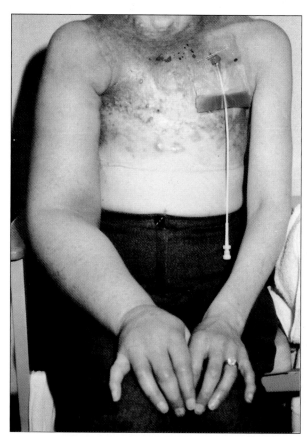

Figure 4.3 Lymphoedema and recurrent disease in 70 year old woman previously treated for breast cancer by means of surgery and radiotherapy

---

Cornerstones of treating lymphoedema (SETS)

- **S**kin care
- **E**xercise and movement
- **T**runcal massage
- **S**upport bandaging or hosiery

500 mg every 6 hours or co-amoxiclav 250/125 mg every 8 hours will clear the infection within days. For patients allergic to penicillin, erythromycin seems equally effective.

With repeated infections, patients should have a supply of antibiotics at home to take at the first sign of infection. Some patients need to take antibiotics for several months (penicillin V 500 mg daily). A few patients have a severe attack with fever, and initial treatment for these patients should be parenteral penicillin or erythromycin.

Fungal infection should be considered; topical antifungal drugs are then indicated.

Skin care

Skin care is essential to reduce the risk of cellulitis. Dry skin should be moisturised and skin breaks dressed with antiseptic cream. An infective dermatitis that is weeping needs soaking with potassium permanganate solution. Persistent leakage of fluid suggests lymphorrhoea, which is most effectively treated by an intensive one to two weeks of massage and bandaging as described below. Before bandaging wet skin, a non-adherent dressing should be applied and the bandaging changed daily or more often if it becomes soaked.

Reducing lymphoedema

Is ischaemia present? If the ratio of posterior tibial artery pressure to brachial artery pressure (measured with Doppler ultrasound scanning) is 0.8 or less, bandages or compression hosiery should not be used.

Is venous obstruction present? If the oedema has occurred within days, venous obstruction by thrombosis or tumour must be excluded.

Is massage possible? This is possible unless the trunk skin is extensively affected by infection, tumour, or other disease. Massage starts in a trunk quadrant free of lymphoedema before moving to the lymphoedematous side. The massage is done gently by hand or electrical massager, and no talc or oil is used. The aim is to move lymph from a lymphoedematous area to one that is clear of lymphoedema. Twice daily massage for about 20 minutes by the patient or carer is sufficient for most lymphoedema.

Is there time to reduce lymphoedema? It takes at least a month to achieve a satisfactory reduction. If a patient's life expectancy is less than this, treatment is unchanged but the aim is to make the patient comfortable and to prevent worsening of the affected area.

Is the lymphoedema midline? Massage alone is used, although for genital and perineal lymphoedema, made to measure pants, tights, or scrotal supports can also be used.

Is support indicated? If bandages are indicated these should be made from high compression, low stretch materials and applied to give a graduated pressure that is highest distally. The bandages are usually applied daily in a single layer but can be applied in several layers for more resistant lymphoedema. With hosiery, tubular supports must be avoided as they often roll and worsen lymphoedema. Class 1-3 hosiery can be prescribed in the community, but many patients require higher compressions, which are available only through hospital prescriptions. Made to measure hosiery is not usually necessary or practical, but it is useful in the few patients with unusually shaped limbs.

Compression pumps are of limited value and should be restricted to those few patients who have no oedema of the nearest trunk quadrant.

Key questions in managing lymphoedema

- Is infection present?
- Is skin drier or wetter than usual?
- Is ischaemia present?
- Is venous obstruction present?
- Is massage possible?
- Will patient's prognosis allow reduction of lymphoedemia?
- Is lymphoedema in midline only?
- Is support indicated?

Support bandaging hosiery

Bandaging	**Hosiery**
Indications	*Indications*
• Fragile or damaged skin	• Intact skin
• Limb too large to fit hosiery	• Patient able to fit and remove it
• Distorted limb shape	
• Pain in site of lymphoedema	• Limb size and shape allow fitting
Contraindications	
• Ratio of posterior tibial: branchial artery pressures < 0.8	*Contraindications and cautions*
• Ventricular failure	• As for bandaging
• Recent peripheral vein thrombosis	
Caution with	
• Microcirculatory problems	
• Absence of sensation	

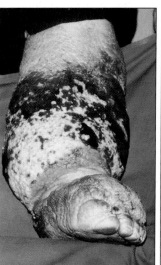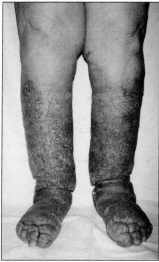

Figure 4.4 Even large volumes of lymphoedema can be reduced with massage and support: 13 litres were removed from the leg shown left to achieve the result shown right. In uncomplicated lymphoedema 40–60% reductions in volume can be cost effectively achieved and maintained for years

5 Nausea, vomiting, and intestinal obstruction

Mary J Baines

Nausea and vomiting

Nausea, vomiting, and retching are common and distressing complaints: surveys have found that 50-60% of patients with advanced cancer suffer from one or more of these. These symptoms are more common in patients under 65 years old, in women, and in those with cancer of the stomach or breast.

Assessment

An understanding of the emetic process and the main neurotransmitters involved is helpful in assessing and treating patients who are vomiting because antiemetic drugs are predominately neurotransmitter blocking agents. They are effective at different receptor sites and therefore treat different causes of vomiting.

As well as the specific causes of vomiting resulting directly or indirectly from advanced malignancy, patients may develop unrelated conditions such as gastroenteritis or gall bladder disease. In most cases the cause of vomiting is multifactorial, but it is helpful in planning treatment to list all contributing factors.

The causes of vomiting can usually be determined from a careful history and clinical examination. Note should be taken of the volume, content, and timing of vomits. A biochemical profile may be needed, but other investigations are often inappropriate.

Management

Nausea can be treated with oral drugs, but alternative routes are needed for patients with severe vomiting. It must be remembered, however, that persistent nausea may decrease gastric emptying, with a resultant decrease in drug absorption. An antiemetic injection is suitable to control a single episode, but with a persistent problem it is preferable to give drugs by subcutaneous infusion using an infusion device such as a pocket sized syringe driver. Antiemetics, in suppository or tablet form, can also be given rectally, but buccal administration of antiemetics is poorly tolerated.

Non-drug methods are important; these include avoidance of food smells or unpleasant odours, diversion, and relaxation. Some patients report benefit from acupuncture or acupressure bands.

Specific cause of vomiting
In a few patients, a specific cause of vomiting can be identified and treated successfully. However, most patients have irreversible and multiple causes of vomiting and require treatment with antiemetics and other measures.

Opioid induced vomiting—About 30% of patients who receive morphine feel nauseated during the first week of treatment. Metoclopramide should be given prophylactically to cover this period. Haloperidol is an alternative.

Cytotoxic chemotherapy—The use of ondansetron, granisetron, or tropisetron—the 5-HT$_3$ receptor antagonists—has greatly improved the control of emesis, even with cisplatin. This effect is enhanced by combining the antiemetic with dexamethasone. High dose metoclopramide and dexamethasone is a less effective but cheaper alternative. Lorazepam is used to reduce anticipatory anxiety and nausea.

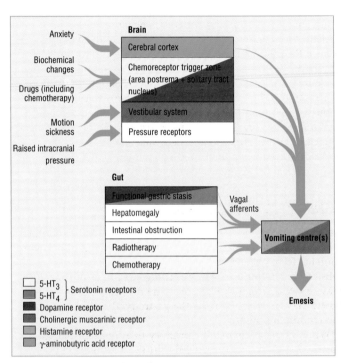

Figure 5.1 The emetic process–pathways of emesis and the neurotransmitters involved

Common causes of vomiting in patients with advanced cancer

- Drugs
    Especially opioids and chemotherapy
- Gastric causes
    Gastritis or ulceration
    Functional gastric stasis
    External pressure
    Carcinoma of stomach
    Gastroduodenal obstruction
- Constipation
- Intestinal obstruction
- Biochemical causes
    Renal failure
    Hypercalcaemia
    Infection
    Tumour toxins
- Raised intracranial pressure
- Vestibular disturbance
- Abdominal or pelvic radiotherapy
- Anxiety
- Cough induced

Reversible causes of vomiting

Causes of vomiting	Treatment
Hypercalcaemia	Rehydration and bisphosphonates
Infection	Antibiotics
Raised intracranial pressure	Dexamethasone
Gastric irritation or ulceration	Stop non-steroidal anti-inflammatory drug Give omeprazole or H$_2$ receptor antagonist
Constipation	Rectal measures and laxatives
Anxiety	Explanation and reassurance, possibly also anxiolytic drugs

Renal failure—Haloperidol is usually effective, although methotrimeprazine is sometimes required for intractable vomiting.

Functional gastric stasis—A prokinetic drug such as metoclopramide, domperidone, or cisapride should be used. The action of these drugs will be blocked by the concomitant use of anticholinergic drugs

Inoperable gastroduodenal obstruction—Metoclopramide may be effective if the obstruction is partial. Dexamethasone was thought to shrink inflammatory oedema around an obstructive lesion, but it may work by reducing perineuronal oedema in a functional obstruction; its antiemetic effect may also be of benefit. Octreotide or high dose hyoscine butylbromide may reduce the volume of vomit, otherwise intubation will be required.

Raised intracranial pressure—If dexamethasone is contraindicated or ineffective, cyclizine is the antiemetic of choice.

Vestibular disturbance—Cyclizine is usually effective, but an alternative is sublingual or transdermal hyoscine hydrobromide.

Intestinal obstruction

Intestinal obstruction is caused by an occlusion to the lumen or a lack of normal propulsion that prevents or delays intestinal contents from passing along the gastrointestinal tract. Obstruction may cause the presenting symptoms of cancer, or may develop during the course of the disease. Any site in the bowel may be affected, from the gastroduodenal junction to the rectum and anus.

While surgery remains the primary treatment for malignant obstruction, it is now recognised that some patients with advanced disease or poor general condition are unfit for surgery and require alternative management to relieve distressing symptoms.

Aetiology
The overall incidence of intestinal obstruction in patients with advanced cancer is about 3%, but patients with advanced ovarian cancer have a risk of obstruction of 25-40%. Patients with metastatic abdominal or pelvic cancer often have both mechanical and functional causes for obstruction, which may occur at more than one site.

Assessment

Clinical features
The symptoms of intestinal obstruction will depend on the site of the problem, a high obstruction causing more severe vomiting. In patients with advanced disease the onset of obstruction is usually insidious, over some weeks. Symptoms may gradually worsen and become continuous, but even without treatment the symptoms may be intermittent and the obstructive episodes resolve spontaneously, if temporarily.

A distinction is often made between complete and partial obstruction, but this is far from easy in practice and, clinically, the obstruction may seem to alter from one type to the other on several occasions as the illness progresses.

Investigations
Radiological investigations are of value in only two clinical situations: firstly, to differentiate between constipation and malignant obstruction; and, secondly, to confirm the obstruction and determine its site and nature in a patient who is being considered for surgery.

Recommended antiemetic drugs

Antiemetic	Dose (per 24 hours)*	Main site of action
Prokinetic		
Metoclopramide†	30-80 mg	Increase peristalsis in upper gut, also dopamine antagonists
Domperidone	30-80 mg	
Cisapride	20-30 mg	Increase peristalsis in gut
Antihistamines		
Cyclizine†	150 mg	Vestibular and vomiting centres
Butyrophenones		
Haloperidol†	1.5-10 mg	Blocks dopamine receptors at chemoreceptor trigger zone
Phenothiazines		
Methotrimeprazine†	12.5-75 mg	Blocks dompamine and serotonin receptors (5-HT$_2$) at chemoreceptor trigger zone, also acts at vestibular and vomiting centres
5-HT$_3$ receptor antagonists		
Ondansetron†	8-16 mg	Blocks 5-HT$_3$ receptors at area postrema and in gut
Granisetron	3 mg	
Corticosteroids		
Dexamethasone†	8-20 mg	Reduces inflammatory oedema, also central and peripheral antiemetic effects
Anticholinergics		
Hyoscine butylbromide†	60-200 mg	Reduces gastrointestinal sectretions and motility
Somatostatin analogues		
Octreotide†	300-600 µg	Reduces gastrointestinal secretions and motility

*A single dose will be a third of the lower dose in the range
†Can be given by subcutaneous infusion

Causes of intestinal obstruction in advanced cancer
- Extrinsic compression from enlargement of primary tumour, omental masses, malignant adhesions, post-irradiation fibrosis
- Intraluminal occlusion from annular tumour or polypoid lesions
- Motility disorders due to tumour infiltration of mesentery or bowel muscle (intestinal linitis plastica)

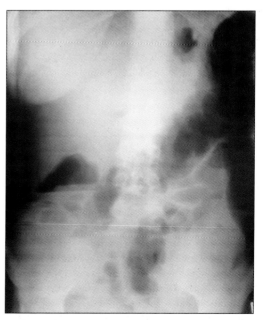

Figure 5.2 Radiograph showing obstruction

ABC of palliative care

Management

There are now several treatment options for patients with advanced cancer who develop intestinal obstruction. It is rarely an emergency, so there is usually time to discuss the situation with patients and their family so that they can make an informed choice of the available treatments.

Palliative surgery

Palliative surgery should be considered for every patient with advanced cancer who develops intestinal obstruction. Some will have a non-malignant cause or an unrelated second primary tumour. However, mortality is high (12-30%), the mean survival time is short, and there is a high incidence of enterocutaneous fistulae.

Nasogastric intubation

This leads to a sustained relief of obstruction in only 0-2% of patients. It should therefore be used only for patients who are being considered for surgery and for those, principally with a high obstruction, who respond poorly to drug treatment. In this group, percutaneous venting gastrostomy should be considered as a better tolerated alternative. This can be performed under local anaesthesia.

Pharmacological treatment

Drugs have been used for years to relieve symptoms, and treatment regimens have gradually evolved. Continuous subcutaneous infusion is the preferred route of drug administration. This allows a combination of drugs to be given, and it is ideal for use in the home as it can be renewed every 24 hours by the visiting nurse.

The symptoms of colic, continuous abdominal pain, and vomiting usually occur together, and a typical starting prescription would be

- Diamorphine (dose depending on previous opioid dose)
- Hyoscine butylbromide 60 mg/24 hours
- Haloperidol 5 mg/24 hours.

If continuous pain or colic is not controlled, the dose of diamorphine or hyoscine butylbromide should be increased. If nausea and vomiting remain problems, cyclizine can be substituted for haloperidol or the two drugs can be used in combination. A useful alternative to this is methotrimeprazine, a highly effective antiemetic in this situation. However, if this fails, and especially if the total volume of vomits is large, octreotide is often used. It is antisecretory, proabsorbtive, and reduces forward peristalsis. It can be combined with other drugs for subcutaneous infusion.

Corticosteroids have been widely used with apparent benefit to individual patients, but, with the intermittent nature of the early symptoms, it is difficult to know if the improvement is due to the corticosteroid treatment.

All patients will need regular mouth care. With good or moderate control of nausea and vomiting, patients can eat and drink as they choose, most favouring small and low residue meals.

A small group of patients, mainly with high obstruction, continue to vomit profusely in spite of medication. These may benefit from the insertion of a nasogastric tube or venting gastrostomy. The need for parenteral hydration should be decided on an individual basis; if indicated, fluids can be given by intravenous infusion or by hypodermoclysis (subcutaneous fluids). This is well tolerated and can be administered in the home supervised by the family and community nursing staff.

Symptoms of intestinal obstruction

- Nausea and vomiting
- Continuous abdominal pain
- Constipation
- Intestinal colic
- Distension
- Diarrhoea (with partial obstruction)

Treatment options in obstruction

- Palliative surgery
- Pharmacological treatment
- Nasogastric intubation
- Percutaneous venting gastrostomy

Factors associated with poor prognosis for palliative surgery

- Aged over 70 years, poor general medical condition or nutritional status
- Ascites, palpable abdominal masses, or distant metastases
- Previous radiotherapy to abdomen or pelvis
- Previous combination chemotherapy
- Multiple small bowel obstructions with radiographic evidence of prolonged transit time

---

Drugs used to relieve symptoms in intestinal obstruction

Drug	Dose (per 24 hours)	Comment
Nausea and vomiting		
Haloperidol	5-10 mg	Antiemetic of choice
Cyclizine	100-150 mg	May crystallise in infusion device
Methotrimeprazine	12.5-75 mg	Highly effective antiemetic Sedating at higher doses
Hyoscine butylbromide	60-200 mg	Reduces gastrointestinal secretions and motility
Octreotide	300-600 µg	Reduces gastrointestinal secretions and motility Expensive
Intestinal colic		
Diamorphine	As required	Usually an antispasmodic is also used
Hyoscine butylbromide	60-200 mg	Not sedating
Continuous abdominal pain		
Diamorphine	As required	
Diarrhoea (from incomplete obstruction or faecal fistula)		
Loperamide	6-16 mg (orally)	
Octreotide	300-600 µg	

6 Anorexia, cachexia, and nutrition

Eduardo Bruera

Cachexia is a complex syndrome that combines weight loss, lipolysis, loss of muscle and visceral protein, anorexia, chronic nausea, and weakness. Severe cachexia occurs in most patients with advanced cancer or AIDS. This article covers approaches to cachexia other than treatment of the underlying disease. In those patients who are eligible for tumouricidal treatment, cachexia may resolve as the disease responds.

When faced with a cachectic patient, the clinician may approach the problem with four questions:
- Does the patient have cachexia?
- Why is the patient cachectic?
- Which treatments are effective?
- How should treatment be individualised?

Does the patient have cachexia?

Frequency of cachexia
More than 80% of patients with cancer or AIDS develop cachexia before death. At the moment of diagnosis, about 80% of patients with upper gastrointestinal cancers and 60% of patients with lung cancer have substantial weight loss. In general, patients with solid tumours (with the exception of breast cancer) have a higher frequency of cachexia. Cachexia is also more common in children and elderly patients and becomes more pronounced as disease progresses.

Assessing nutritional status
Because of the chronic nature of cancer cachexia, the diagnosis is simple. A patient's clinical history, the presence of substantial weight loss, and physical examination are adequate for an accurate diagnosis.

Plasma albumin concentration is usually decreased. Simple bedside measurements—such as triceps or subscapular skin folds (for body fat) and arm muscular circumference (for body lean mass)—may be useful to monitor nutritional changes or the effect of treatments in patients in whom body weight might be unreliable (such as those with ascites or oedema).

More sophisticated laboratory investigations are usually unnecessary. Immunological tests are unreliable markers of nutritional status in patients with cancer or AIDS because of the immunological abnormalities due to the underlying illness.

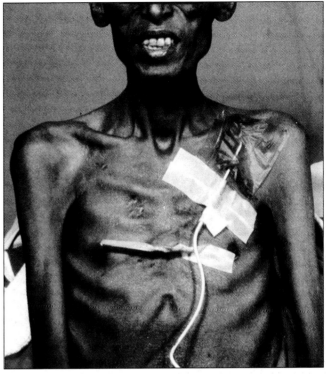

Figure 6.1   Patient with cachexia

Effects of cachexia
- Decreased survival
- Increased complications of surgery, radiotherapy, and chemotherapy
- Weakness, anorexia, chronic nausea
- Psychological distress in patient and family

Why is the patient cachectic?

While metabolic abnormalities are the main cause of malnutrition, decreased caloric intake and malabsorption also contribute to the cachexia syndrome.

Decreased caloric intake
Anorexia is an almost universal component of cachexia. Reduced caloric intake may be more severe in patients with dysphagia due to head and neck pain or oesophageal carcinoma, psychological depression, abnormalities of taste, or chronic nausea. The last is a common symptom in malignant diseases and can be due to autonomic failure, opioids and other drugs, constipation, or bowel obstruction.

> In most patients cachexia is caused by metabolic abnormalities due to the production of tumour products and cytokines by the immune system. Anorexia is a major contributor to cachexia in a minority of patients, but in most it is simply a symptom of cachexia

Metabolic abnormalities

Traditionally, cancer was assumed to cause cachexia by consuming energy and by releasing factors capable of causing anorexia. This interpretation justified aggressive nutrition as an approach to restore the energy balance.

The emerging view is that cachexia of cancer is mainly due to major metabolic abnormalities. These are caused predominantly by cytokines released by the immune system as a response to the presence of the cancer (cachectin-tumour necrosis factor and interleukins 1 and 6) and are probably also related to the cachexia of other diseases such as AIDS, tuberculosis, and leprosy.

Tumour products have also been identified (such as lipolytic hormones). These factors cause profound lipolysis, negative nitrogen balance, and anorexia. In most patients, anorexia is more likely the result of the catabolic process rather than the cause of the cachexia. This view explains the failure of aggressive nutrition in changing clinical outcome, symptoms, and the nutritional status of cancer patients.

Malabsorption

This should be suspected in patients with pancreatic insufficiency due to pancreatic or other gastrointestinal cancers, or in patients who have recently received aggressive radiation therapy to the abdomen. It is an uncommon cause of malnutrition.

Which treatments are effective?

Weight loss is an independent risk factor for poor survival. Cachectic patients have a higher incidence of complications after surgery, radiotherapy, and chemotherapy. In addition, cachexia aggravates weakness, is associated with anorexia and chronic nausea, and is a source of psychological distress for patients and families because of the associated symptoms and the changes in body image. This prompts some to attempt aggressive nutritional supplementation.

Advantages of intensive nutrition

The complications of cachexia and the view that it results mostly from an energy deficit has generated many studies attempting to reverse these complications with total parenteral or enteral nutrition. Unfortunately, these studies have generally found no significant improvement in patient survival or tumour shrinkage, and limited effects on the complications associated with surgery, radiotherapy, or chemotherapy. Since most studies failed to assess patients' symptoms it is not clear if intensive nutrition confers any symptomatic benefits.

However, intensive nutrition is appropriate in certain clinical situations, such as in patients recovering from surgery and awaiting chemotherapy. When selecting patients for nutrition, doctors must take into account the morbidity (15% in some studies) and the financial cost.

Effects of pharmacological management

Several drugs have beneficial effects on the symptoms of cachexia, and some have effects on patients' nutritional status.

Corticosteroids

These improve both anorexia and weakness in cancer patients. However, these effects are purely subjective and are not accompanied by any important improvement in caloric intake or nutritional status. The effects are usually short lasting (limited to 3-4 weeks), but they are usually well tolerated for brief periods even in very ill patients.

Probable causes of cachexia

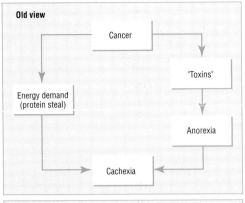

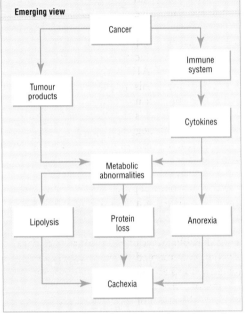

Figure 6.2 Traditional and emerging views of causes of cancer cachexia

---

Therapeutic options

- Dietry advice
- Nutritional supplementation
- Prokinetic drugs
- Corticosteroids
- Progestational drugs
- Tumouricidal treatment (if appropriate)

An identifiable and reversible cause of weight loss is an indication for intensive nutrition

---

Effects of intensive nutrition

- No increase in survival
- No improved tumour shrinkage
- Minimal decrease in toxicity of chemotherapy or radiotherapy
- Minimal decrease in surgical morbidity
- Unknown symptomatic effects

The mechanism of action is unknown but is possibly related to inhibition of the release of metabolic products by the tumour or immune system or to a non-specific central euphoriant effect.

Corticosteroids also have antiemetic and other effects, including analgesia, improvement in neurological symptoms due to cerebral oedema and spinal cord or nerve compression, decrease in breathlessness due to lymphangitis carcinomatosis, and anecdotal reports of a beneficial effect on the symptoms associated with bowel and ureteral obstruction.

Progestational drugs

Medroxyprogesterone and megestrol acetate may substantially improve appetite, caloric intake, and nutritional status in patients with advanced cancer or AIDS. These drugs also result in an increased deposition of fat. Controlled trials have shown that megestrol acetate improves several symptoms in addition to appetite, including a sensation of wellbeing, reduced fatigue, and some aspects of quality of life. When used as an appetite stimulant, megestrol acetate has no effect on survival of patients with cancer or AIDS.

The progestational drugs' mechanism of action is unclear. Since intensive nutrition has limited nutritional effects and no obvious symptomatic advantages, it is unlikely that both the subjective and objective effects of megestrol acetate are due to increased appetite and caloric intake. More likely, these drugs have an effect on the metabolic abnormalities due to the cancer, and the increase in appetite is secondary to reversal of the catabolic state. The main drawback of progestogens is their high cost and side effects such as oedema and thrombotic episodes.

Prokinetic agents

These can have a considerable effect on symptoms in patients complaining of anorexia accompanied by early satiety or chronic nausea. Such symptoms are mostly due to gastroparesis because of autonomic failure, brought on by the presence of the cancer or malnutrition, or the effect of drugs such as opioids or tricyclic antidepressants.

Other drugs

Other drugs are thought to have effects on appetite, but the evidence is anecdotal and clinical use is not justified at this time. Clinical trials are being conducted on cyproheptadine, oxpentifylline, melatonin, thalidomide, certain cannabinoids, and low doses of alcohol.

Hydrazine sulfate has had publicity in north America and is used widely as an 'alternative' drug for cancer cachexia. Three recent randomised controlled trials have found it no more effective than placebo with regards to nutritional status, survival, symptoms of cachexia, or quality of life. In addition, it causes considerable toxicity, including peripheral neuropathy.

Work on fish oil extract if showing promise.

Individualising treatment

Determining expectations and outcomes

It is extremely important to establish initially what patients, their family, and their physician expect from any treatment. Neither nutritional nor drug treatments confer any survival advantage in metastatic cancer. Intensive nutritional replacement has limited, if any, value for patients with advanced and progressive disease; exceptions may include head and neck tumours that advance locally but metastasise slowly and neurological disorders such as motor neurone disease.

Although megestrol acetate and, in some cases, artificial nutrition provide nutritional improvement, this alone does not justify treatments that are potentially toxic for terminally ill patients unless there is a substantial benefit to quality of life.

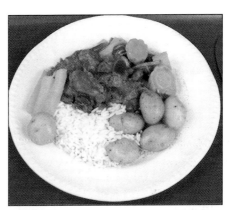

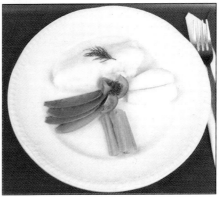

Figure 6.3 The size and appearance of meals may be as important as their nutritional value. Standard hospital meals (top) are generally unsuitable and should be replaced by smaller, more attractive helpings (bottom)

Choice of treatment

Nutritional counselling should be based on eating high calorie meals of small portions that are pleasant for the patient. It is important to include the patient's family in such discussions. It is useful to clarify that an excess of calories is unlikely to benefit the patient by explaining that his or her metabolic system does not have the ability to use these calories in the same way as that of a healthy person. Although cachectic, the patient is not "starving."

Patients who are unable to swallow because of severe dysphagia (for example, because of head and neck or oesophageal cancers and neurological disorders) and who complain of hunger or express concerns related to malnutrition may benefit from nutrition via a gastrostomy tube. Such tubes can be inserted with ultrasonographic or endoscopic guidance.

Patients with chronic nausea, early satiety, or other findings suggesting gastroparesis should receive a trial of a prokinetic drug. Patients with slowly progressive illness for whom anorexia is an important symptom may benefit from both the symptomatic and nutritional effects of megestrol acetate. Severely ill patients with multiple complex symptoms and a limited life expectancy are more likely to benefit from the multiple symptomatic effects of a course of corticosteroids. Finally, patients for whom anorexia is a relatively minor problem or those who are severely cognitively impaired may not require any treatment.

In patients with mechanical bowel obstruction, prokinetic drugs may aggravate emesis. Antiemetics, octreotide, hyoscine, or nasogastric drainage will be required for symptom relief. Some special conditions may further reduce food intake and require assessment and management; these include chemotherapy or radiotherapy induced mucositis or emesis and severe depression.

Future developments

Clinical trials are currently being conducted on drugs with a subjective effect on appetite and energy, anabolic agents, and drugs capable of inhibiting the release of cachectin-tumour necrosis factor. Differential nutrition with amino acids and fatty acids capable of influencing the metabolic response of the tumour are also being investigated.

Choosing treatments for cachexia

- Intensive nutrition is expensive, associated with morbidity, and there is limited evidence that it can reverse these problems
- Corticosteroids and megestrol acetate are effective appetite stimulants. The weight gain associated with megestrol acetate takes some weeks to manifest
- Prokinetic drugs may improve nausea and early satiety
- The psychological aspects of cachexia can be the most important for patients and their carers. Feeding a dependant is the essence of nature and this fundamental breakdown must be addressed. Explanations and practical solutions are often more important than any drugs administered

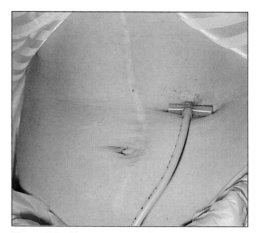

Figure 6.4   Percutaneous endoscopic gastrostomy

7 Constipation and diarrhoea

Marie Fallon, Bill O'Neill

Prevalence of constipation

Constipation can be defined as the passage of small hard faeces infrequently and with difficulty. Constipation is more common in patients with advanced cancer than in those with other terminal diseases, and many of the associated symptoms may mimic features of the underlying disease. About half of patients admitted to specialist palliative care units report constipation, but about 80% of patients will require laxatives.

Assessment of constipation

History

An accurate history is essential for effective management. Inquiry should be made about the frequency and consistency of stools, nausea, vomiting, abdominal pain, distention and discomfort, mobility, diet, and any other symptoms. In patients with a history of diarrhoea, care should be taken to distinguish true diarrhoea from overflow due to faecal impaction.

Careful questioning about access to a toilet or commode is important. Limited mobility may mean that using the toilet or commode is avoided. Other issues, such as lack of privacy or the need for nurses or carers to help with toileting, can exacerbate constipation.

Examination

A constipated patient may have malodorous breath, or the smell of faecal leakage may be obvious. Bacterial degradation of hard stools can result in leakage, of which the patient has no warning. General observation may reveal that a patient is in pain, confused or disorientated, or unable to reach the toilet. Abdominal distension, visible peristalsis, and borborygmi can suggest obstruction.

Palpation may reveal an easily palpable colon with indentable and mobile (and rarely tender) faecal masses. In contrast, tumour masses are usually hard, not indentable, fixed, and often tender. In constipation complicated by obstruction, auscultation of the abdomen may reveal high pitched tinkling bowel sounds, although the abdomen can also be silent.

Digital examination of the rectum or stoma is crucial if constipation is suspected—this will immediately reveal hard stools, tumour masses, or concomitant disease such as haemorrhoids, an anal fissure, or perianal ulceration. The rectum or stoma can be empty in constipation—hard or even impacted stools can lie higher in the bowel.

Constipation may herald a spinal cord compression. If a neurological deficit is suspected a full neurological examination is essential, including assessment of sphincter tone and rectal sensation. Referral, if appropriate, should be made as an emergency.

Investigation

Occasionally, despite an accurate history and examination, the diagnosis of constipation is still not clear. A plain *x* ray of the abdomen can be useful. Large amounts of stools may appear as clumps of rounded masses with entrapped gas and varying degrees of dilated bowel. Rarely, toxic dilation of the colon may be seen.

Constipation

Definition
- Infrequent hard stools

Associated symptoms
- Flatulence
- Bloating
- Abdominal pain
- Feeling of incomplete evacuation

Symptoms of complications
- Anorexia
- Overflow diarrhoea
- Confusion
- Nausea and vomiting
- Urinary dysfunction

> Assessment of constipation must include establishing in what way the present pattern of bowel movements is different from the normal pattern and a physical examination, including general observation, abdominal palpation, and rectal or stomal examination

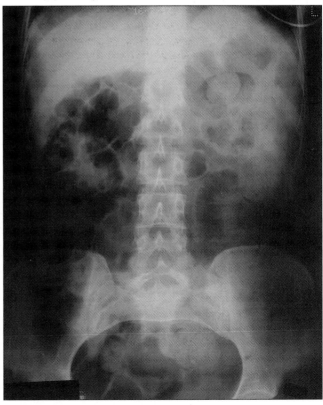

Figure 7.1   Radiograph of constipated patient showing masses and trapped gas

Causes of constipation

Knowledge of the underlying cause helps in both prophylaxis and treatment. The most important of these are immobility, poor fluid and dietary intake, and drugs, particularly opioids.

Opioid induced constipation

In patients with cancer and pain, the use of opioids is the commonest cause of constipation, particularly in immobile patients. Opioids cause constipation by maintaining or increasing intestinal smooth muscle tone, by suppressing forward peristalsis, by raising sphincter tone at the ileocaecal valve and anal sphincter, and by reducing sensitivity to rectal distension. This results in delayed passage of faeces through the gut, with resultant increase in absorption of electrolytes and water in the small intestine and colon.

Gastrointestinal obstruction

Sometimes, a combination of hard stools in the bowel and intrinsic or extrinsic bowel tumour or pelvic tumour coexist, causing gastrointestinal obstruction. With appropriate management of the constipation, the obstructive symptoms may resolve (intestinal obstruction has been covered in an earlier article in this series).

Neurological problems

Bowel management is particularly troublesome and is a common problem in patients with spinal cord compression or cauda equina syndrome. A combination of immobility, loss of rectal sensation, poor anal and colonic tone, and pain may result in constipation with overflow and variable degrees of abdominal distension, nausea, and vomiting.

A cauda equina lesion will abolish the anocolonic reflex, but a higher spinal cord lesion leaves this reflex intact. In the latter case, digital rectal stimulation or suppositories will stimulate colonic contraction and aid evacuation of the colon, whereas in the cauda equina syndrome the colon remains lax.

The aim in managing spinal cord compression or cauda equina syndrome is to attain a "controlled continence." This means giving an individualised combination of oral laxatives daily with suppositories or enemas every two to three days to enable rectal evacuation. The intention is to avoid incontinence in those patients with loss of rectal sensation.

Managing constipation

The management of constipation extends well beyond the use of laxatives. Attention to other symptoms—especially pain and advice on diet, fluid intake, mobility, and toileting—contributes to an effective outcome.

The aim of laxative therapy is to achieve comfortable defecation, rather than any particular frequency of evacuation. Although most laxatives are not very palatable, oral laxatives should be used whenever possible. The choice of laxative depends on the nature of the stools, the cause of the constipation, and acceptability to the patient. Laxatives can be subdivided into three groups:
- Predominantly softening
- Predominantly peristalsis stimulating
- Combination of the two.

When choosing laxatives, a knowledge of the main mechanism of action of laxatives is helpful. Many of the softeners increase stool bulk and lead to reflex stimulation of peristalsis, and, similarly, the peristalsis stimulators enhance intestinal fluid secretion and therefore improve stool consistency.

Causes of constipation

Caused by cancer	Caused by treatment
● Hypercalcaemia	● Opioids
● Intra-abdominal or pelvic disease	● Antiemetics—cyclizine, ondansetron
● Spinal cord compression	● Anticholinergics—antispasmodics, antidepressants, neuroleptics
● Cauda equina syndrome	● Aluminium salts
● Depression	● Non-steroidal anti-inflammatory drugs

Associated with debility
- Weakness
- Inactivity or bed rest
- Poor nutrition
- Poor fluid intake
- Confusion
- Inability to reach the toilet

Concurrent disorders
- Haemorrhoids
- Anal fissure
- Endocrine dysfunction

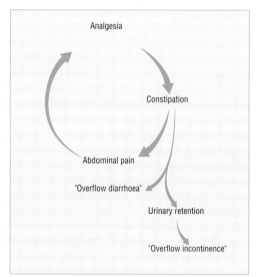

Figure 7.2 Vicious cycle of constipation associated with opioid analgesia

> A distended rectum or colon can be a potent cause of agitation and pain in a dying patient. Evacuation of the rectum or colon with suppositories alone or with an enema can give complete relief of agitation. The use of opioids to treat the pain of constipation only makes the constipation, and ultimately the pain, worse and a vicious cycle ensues

Oral laxatives

Predominantly softening
Surfactants—Sodium docusate, poloxamer
Osmotic laxatives—Lactulose, sorbitol
Bulking agents—Ispaghula, methyl cellulose
Saline laxatives—Magnesium sulphate
Lubricants—Liquid paraffin

Predominantly peristalsis stimulating
Anthracenes—Senna, danthron
Polyphenolics—Bisacodyl, sodium picosulphate

Predominantly softening laxatives

Surfactant laxatives act as detergents, increasing water penetration and hence softening the stools. Docusate also promotes secretion of water, sodium, and chloride in the jejunum and colon. Poloxamer and docusate have a latency of action of one to three days. Docusate is often used alone as a softener in intermittent bowel obstruction. It is also used in combination with the peristalsis stimulator danthron (as co-danthrusate). Poloxamer is marketed only in combination with danthron (co-danthramer). Both co-danthrusate and co-danthramer are effective laxatives for opioid induced constipation.

Osmotic laxatives—The most popular in this group is lactulose. Its latency of action is up to three days. It flushes the small bowel and, with larger doses, tends to result in bloating and colic. Flatulence and its sweet taste can cause problems with compliance. Sorbitol is cheaper and less nauseating. Osmotic laxatives should be accompanied by an increase in fluid intake.

Bulk forming agents are stool normalisers rather than true laxatives. They are less helpful in cancer patients because of the volume of water required, their unproved efficacy in severe constipation, and the possibility of worsening an incipient obstruction.

Saline laxatives—These, especially magnesium sulphate, can produce an undesirably strong purgative action. Magnesium hydroxide is also used in combination with liquid paraffin (Milpar).

Lubricants—Liquid paraffin is now rarely used because of its unpleasant taste and because, with long term use, it can cause considerable irritation. Aspiration can result in a lipoidal pneumonia.

Peristalsis stimulating laxatives

These drugs directly stimulate the myenteric plexus to induce peristalsis and reduce net absorption of water and electrolytes in the colon, making them particularly useful in opioid induced constipation. Their latency of action is 6-12 hours. Any bowel stimulant can cause abdominal colic and severe purgation. The dose of stimulant should be titrated as with any potent drug and consideration given to dose at each administration; colic may be reduced by giving the total daily requirement in divided doses.

Senna can be used in combination with a softener such as lactulose. Equal proportions of senna liquid and lactulose are more potent than standard co-danthramer (danthron and poloxamer), but seem less potent than co-danthramer forte.

Senna and danthron directly counteract the important constipating effects of opioids and can be highly effective when used with a stool softener. They are invaluable in colonic inertias. Patients given danthron should be warned of the pink or red discolouration of the urine, and the perianal area should be watched for a danthron rash, particularly in incontinent patients, who may require a barrier cream.

Rectal laxatives

Rectal laxatives are sometimes necessary but should never accompany an inadequate prescription of an oral laxative. They are necessary for treating faecal impaction and for conditions such as spinal cord compression, when long term use may be necessary. They should not, however, be part of the regular treatment of every cancer patient with constipation. They are undignified and inconvenient and may have a considerable negative effect on quality of life.

Rectal laxatives are available as suppositories or enemas, and their mode of action is similar to that of the equivalent oral agent. Soft stools in a lax rectum can be evacuated by a stimulant such as bisacodyl, and hard stools in the rectum can

---

Formulations of laxatives

Co-danthrusate
Combination of softener (docusate) and stimulant (danthron)
- Capsules—2 capsules at night up to 3 capsules four times daily

Co-danthramer
Combination of softener (poloxamer) and stimulant (danthron); available in standard strength or forte (with 3 times as much danthron as standard but 5 times as much poloxamer)
- Capsules—2 capsules at night up to 3 capsules four times daily
- Liquid—15 ml at night up to 15 ml thrice daily

Lactulose*
Softener
- Liquid—15 ml twice daily (according to patient's needs)

Senna*
Stimulant
- Tablets—2-4 tablets at night (if larger dose, split administration)
- Liquid

Sodium docusate
Softener (useful in intermittent bowel obstruction)
- Tablets—100-200 mg thrice daily
- Liquid—100-200 mg thrice daily

*Often used together

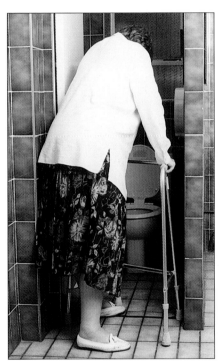

Figure 7.3 Access and ability to get to a lavatory may be more important in constipation than supply of laxatives

---

Questions to guide choice of rectal laxative
- Is the rectum or stoma full?
- Is the stool hard or soft?
- Is the rectum or stoma empty but the colon full?
- Are the rectum and colon both full?
- Does the patient have rectal sensation?
- Does the patient have normal anal tone?
- If a cord lesion is present what is the level?

Choices of rectal laxative

Bisacodyl suppository—Evacuates stools from rectum or stoma; for colonic inertia
Glycerine suppository—Soften stools in rectum or stoma
Phosphate enema—Evacuates stools from lower bowel
Arachis oil enema—Softens hard impacted stools

be softened with glycerine suppositories. A combination of a bisacodyl suppository with a glycerine suppository is sometimes helpful. In cases of colonic inertia, a bisacodyl suppository placed in direct contact with the rectal mucosa may produce rapid results.

Lubricant enemas such as arachis oil are normally given overnight as retention enemas to soften very hard stools in the rectum or higher up, before administration of a saline rectal laxative such as sodium phosphate. In such severe cases the enema should be administered high with a Foley catheter and not just placed in the lower rectum, from where it will leak out as it is administered. The catheter balloon can be inflated for 10 minutes to minimise immediate return of the enema.

For less severe impaction, a high phosphate enema may suffice. Enemas may need to be repeated several times to clear the bowel of hard impacted faeces; patients can then usually be maintained with regular oral laxatives.

When rectal laxatives are required, an appropriate oral laxative should be prescribed at the same time. Once disimpaction occurs, the dose of oral laxative may need to be titrated with the aim of reaching a maintenance dose that prevents further faecal impaction.

Management of constipation in patients with stomas should follow the principles outlined above, but it must be remembered that no sphincter exists. Suppositories should be held in place with a gloved finger, and enemas should be retained by inflating a Foley catheter balloon for 10 minutes.

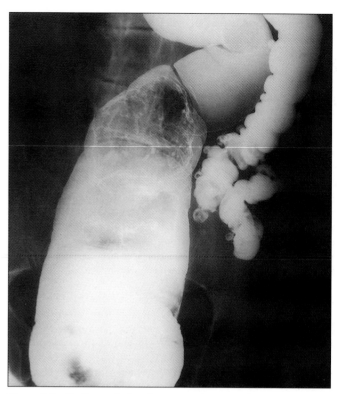

Figure 7.4 Radiograph showing megacolon secondary to rectal impaction

Diarrhoea

With the exception of patients with AIDS, diarrhoea is much less common than constipation in patients with advanced disease. Less than 10% of those with cancer admitted to hospital or palliative care units have diarrhoea. Diarrhoea can be highly debilitating in a patient with advanced disease because of loss of fluid and electrolytes, anxiety about soiling, and the effort of repeatedly going to the lavatory.

Causes

The commonest cause of diarrhoea in patients with advanced disease is use of laxatives. Patients may use laxatives erratically; some wait until they become constipated and then use high doses of laxatives, with resultant rebound diarrhoea. Some patients complain that their laxatives are too strong; adequate explanation on the use of laxatives may solve the problem.

Among elderly patients admitted to hospital with non-malignant disease, constipation with faecal impaction and overflow accounts for over half the cases of diarrhoea. Such patients require rectal laxatives together with a stool softener; care is required with stimulant laxatives as they may cause colic.

Management

Consideration must be given to the underlying cause, but, with the exception of the scenarios above, symptomatic relief is generally achieved with non-specific antidiarrhoeal agents—loperamide (up to 16 mg daily) or codeine (10-60 mg every 4 hours). Codeine may cause central effects such as drowsiness or sedation, but this is rare with loperamide. In general, a single drug should be used, and care should be taken to avoid subtherapeutic doses of combinations of drugs.

Rarely, intractable diarrhoea may require a subcutaneous infusion of octreotide; the usual indication is a high effluent volume from a stoma. Obstructive rectal and pelvic lesions can be managed by radiotherapy and chemotherapy, surgery, stenting or, in the case of rectal lesions, laser therapy. Palliative surgery may be necessary for patients with a fistula.

Causes of diarrhoea in advanced disease

- Drugs
  Laxatives
  Antibiotics
  Antacids
  Chemotherapy (5-fluorouracil)
- Radiotherapy
- Intestinal obstruction (including faecal impaction)
- Concurrent disease, such as inflammatory bowel disease
- Diet
- Tumour
  Colon or rectum
  Pelvic
  Pancreatic (islet cell)
  Carcinoid
  Fistula
- Malabsorption
  Pancreatic carcinoma
  Gastrectomy
  Ileal resection
  Colectomy
- Infection

Specific treatments for diarrhoea

- Cholestyramine
  Radiotherapy induced diarrhoea
  Chologenic diarrhoea
- Ranitidine (or other H$_2$ antagonist)
  Zollinger-Ellison syndrome
  Fat malabsorption (with Pancreatin)
- Cyproheptadine
  Carcinoid syndrome

8 Depression, anxiety, and confusion

Jennifer Barraclough

A common mistake is to assume that depression and anxiety represent nothing more than natural and understandable reactions to incurable illness. When cure is not possible, the analytical approach we adopt to physical and psychological signs and symptoms is often forgotten. Excuse is found in the overlap of symptoms due to physical disease, depression, and anxiety. This error of approach and the lack of diagnostic importance given to major and minor symptoms of depression result in underdiagnosis and treatment of psychiatric disorder.

The emotional and cognitive changes in patients with advanced disease reflect both psychological and biological effects of the medical condition and its treatment. Psychological adjustment reactions after diagnosis or relapse often include fear, sadness, perplexity, and anger. These usually resolve within a few weeks with the help of the patients' own personal resources, family support, and professional care. A minority of patients, about 10-20%, develop formal psychiatric disorders that require specific evaluation and management in addition to general support. It is important to recognise psychiatric disorders because, if untreated, they add to patients' suffering and hamper their ability to come to terms with their illness, put their affairs in order, and communicate with others.

Emotional distress and psychiatric disorder also affect some relatives and staff.

Causes

Depression and anxiety are usually reactions to the losses and threats of the medical illness. Other risk factors often contribute.

Confusion usually reflects an organic mental disorder from one or more causes, often worsened by bewilderment and distress, discomfort or pain, and being in strange surroundings with strange carers. Elderly patients with impaired memory, hearing, or sight are especially at risk. Unfortunately, reversible causes of confusion are underdiagnosed, and this causes unnecessary distress in patients and families.

Clinical features

Depression and anxiety

These are broad terms that cover a continuum of emotional states. It is not always possible on the basis of a single interview to distinguish self limiting distress, which forms a natural part of the adjustment process, from the psychiatric syndromes of depressive illness and anxiety state, which need specific treatment. Borderline cases are common, and both the somatic and psychological symptoms of depression and anxiety can make diagnosis difficult.

Somatic symptoms—These are often the presenting symptoms, and they overlap with symptoms of the physical illness. For example, depression may manifest as intractable pain, while anxiety can manifest as nausea or dyspnoea. Such symptoms may seem disproportionate to the medical pathology and respond poorly to medical treatments.

Psychological symptoms—Although these might seem understandable, they differ in severity, duration, and quality from 'normal' distress. Depressed patients seem to loathe themselves, over and above loathing their disease. This

Losses and threats of major illness
- Knowledge of a life threatening diagnosis, prognostic uncertainty, fears about dying and death
- Physical symptoms such as pain and nausea
- Unwanted effects of medical and surgical treatments
- Loss of functional capacity, loss of independence, enforced changes in role
- Practical issues such as finance, work, housing
- Changes in relationships, concern for dependants
- Changes in body image, sexual dysfunction, infertility

Risk factors for anxiety and depression
- Organic mental disorders
- Poorly controlled physical symptoms
- Poor relationships and communication between staff and patient
- Past history of mood disorder or misuse of alcohol or drugs
- Personality traits hindering adjustment—Such as rigidity, pessimism, extreme need for independence and control
- Concurrent life events or social difficulties
- Lack of support from family and friends

Common causes of organic mental disorders
- Prescribed drugs—Opioids, psychotropic drugs, corticosteroids, some cytotoxic drugs
- Infection—Respiratory or urinary infection, septicaemia
- Macroscopic brain pathology—Primary or secondary tumour, Alzheimer's disease, cerebrovascular disease, HIV dementia
- Metabolic—Dehydration, electrolyte disturbance, hypercalcaemia, organ failure
- Drug withdrawal—Benzodiazepines, opioids, alcohol

Symptoms and signs of depression
Somatic
- Reduced energy, fatigue
- Disturbed sleep, especially early morning waking
- Diminished appetite
- Psychomotor agitation or retardation

Psychological
- Low mood present most of the time, characteristically worse in the morning
- Loss of interest and pleasure
- Reduced concentration and attention
- Indecisiveness
- Feelings of guilt or worthlessness
- Pessimistic or hopeless ideas about the future
- Suicidal thoughts or acts

manifests through guilt about being ill and a burden to others, pervasive loss of interest and pleasure, and hopelessness about the future. Suicide attempts or requests for euthanasia, however rational they might seem, often indicate clinical depression.

Confusion

This may present as forgetfulness, disorientation in time and place, and changes in mood or behaviour. The two main clinical syndromes are dementia (chronic brain syndrome), which is usually permanent, and delirium (acute brain syndrome), which is potentially reversible.

Delirium, which is more relevant to palliative care, comprises clouding of consciousness with various other abnormalities of mental function from an organic cause. Severity often fluctuates, worsening after dark. Paranoid ideas can be exacerbated by the mental mechanisms of "projection" and "denial"—for example, attributing symptoms to poisoned food rather than a progressive illness. Dehydration, neglect of personal hygiene, and accidental self injury may hasten physical and mental decline. Noisy, demanding, or aggressive behaviour may upset or harm other people. So called "terminal anguish" is a combination of delirium and overwhelming anxiety in the last few days of life.

Recognition

Various misconceptions about psychiatric disorders in medical patients contribute to their widespread underrecognition and undertreatment. Education and training in communication skills, for both patients and staff, could help to remedy this.

Standardised screening instruments include the hospital anxiety and depression (HAD) scale for mood disorder and the mini mental state (MMS) or mental status schedule (MSS) for cognitive impairment. Though not sensitive or specific enough to substitute for assessment by interview, they can help to detect unsuspected cases, contribute to diagnostic assessment of probable cases, and provide a baseline for monitoring progress.

Knowledge of previous personality and psychological state is helpful in identifying high risk patients or those with evolving symptoms, and relatives' observations of any recent change should be heeded.

Prevention and management

General guidelines for both prevention and management include providing an explanation about the illness, in the context of ongoing supportive relationships with known and trusted professionals. Patients should have the opportunity to express their feelings without fear of censure or abandonment. This facilitates the process of adjustment, helping patients to move on towards accepting their situation and making the most of their remaining life.

Visits from a specialised palliative care nurse (such as a Macmillan nurse) or attendance at a palliative care day centre, combined with follow up by the primary healthcare team, often benefit both patients and families. Religious or spiritual counselling may be relevant. Psychiatric referral is indicated when emotional disturbances are severe, atypical, or resistant to treatment; when there is concern about suicide; and on the rare occasions when compulsory measures under the Mental Health Act 1983 seem to be indicated.

Non-drug therapies, both "mainstream" and "complementary," share the common features of increasing patients' sense of participation and control, providing interest and occupation when jobs or hobbies have had to be discontinued, and offering a supportive personal relationship.

Symptoms and signs of anxiety

Psychological
- Apprehension, worry, inability to relax
- Difficulty in concentrating, irritability
- Difficulty falling asleep, unrefreshing sleep, nightmares

Motor tension
- Muscular aches and fatigue
- Restlessness, trembling, jumpiness
- Tension headaches

Autonomic
- Shortness of breath, palpitations, lightheadedness, dizziness
- Sweating, dry mouth, 'lump in throat'
- Nausea, diarrhoea, urinary frequency

Symptoms and signs of delirium
- Clouding of consciousness (reduced awareness of environment)
- Impaired attention
- Impaired memory, especially recent memory
- Impaired abstract thinking and comprehension
- Disorientation in time, place, or person
- Perceptual distortions—Illusions and hallucinations, usually visual or tactile
- Transient delusions, usually paranoid
- Psychomotor disturbance—Agitation or underactivity
- Disturbed cycle of sleeping and waking, nightmares
- Emotional disturbance—Depression, anxiety, fear, irritability, euphoria, apathy, perplexity

---

Underrecognition of psychiatric disorders
- Patients reluctant to voice emotional complaints—Fear of seeming weak or ungrateful; stigma
- Professionals reluctant to inquire—Lack of time, lack of skill, emotional self protection
- Attributing somatic symptoms to medical illness
- Assuming emotional distress is inevitable and untreatable

References for screening instruments

Hospital anxiety and depression scale—Zigmond AS, Snaith RP. The hospital anxiety and depression (HAD) scale. *Acta Psychiatr Scand* 1983;67:361-70

Mini mental state—Folstein MF, Folstein SE, McHugh PR. "Mini-Mental State"—a practical method of grading the cognitive state of patients for the clinician. *J Psychiatr Res* 1975;12:189-98

Mental status schedule—Hodkinson HM. Evaluation of a mental test score for assessment of mental impairment in the elderly. *Age Ageing* 1972;1:233-8

Principles of psychological management
- Sensitive breaking of bad news
- Providing information in accord with individual wishes
- Permitting expression of emotion
- Clarification of concerns and problems
- Patient involved in making decisions about treatment
- Setting realistic goals
- Appropriate package of medical, psychological, and social care
- Continuity of care from named staff

Usually delivered in regular planned sessions, they can also help in acute situations—for example, deep breathing, relaxation techniques, or massage for acute anxiety or panic attacks.

For bedridden patients who are anxious or confused as well as very sick, it is important to provide nursing care from a few trusted people; a quiet, familiar, safe, and comfortable environment; explanation of any practical procedure in advance; and an opportunity to discuss underlying fears.

Relatives also need explanation and support.

Psychotropic drugs

For more severe cases, drug treatment is indicated in addition to, not instead of, the general measures described above.

Depression

Drugs should be prescribed if a definite depressive syndrome is present or if a depressive adjustment reaction fails to resolve within a few weeks. The antidepressant effect of all these drugs may be delayed for several weeks after starting therapy.

Tricyclic antidepressants produce a worthwhile response in about 80% of patients, and their sedative, anxiolytic, and analgesic properties may bring added benefits. However, they have considerable anticholinergic side effects, and they are toxic in overdose. Amitriptyline is the standard compound; dothiepin is similar but is sometimes better tolerated. For both drugs, low doses in the range 25-50 mg at night are sometimes effective, but many patients need 75-150 mg or more. Lofepramine, at doses of 70-210 mg daily, has lower toxicity.

Specific serotonin reuptake inhibitors such as sertraline (50 mg daily) or paroxetine (20 mg daily) have few anticholinergic effects, are non-sedative, and are safe in overdose. However, they may cause nausea, diarrhoea, headache, or anxiety. Several newer related antidepressants have recently become available.

Other treatments—Many alternative compounds are also available, and the less widely used ones—including monoamine oxidase inhibitors, psychostimulants, lithium, and various combinations of antidepressants—may be tried on psychiatric advice with due regard to their interactions with other drugs. For severe depression only, electroconvulsive therapy is safe and rapidly effective. Organic mental disorders do not necessarily contraindicate the use of antidepressant drugs or electroconvulsive therapy.

Anxiety

Benzodiazepines are best limited to short term or intermittent use; prolonged administration may lead to a decline in anxiolytic effect, and cumulative psychomotor impairment. Low dose neuroleptic drugs such as haloperidol 1.5-5 mg daily are an alternative. ß blockers are useful for autonomic overactivity. Chronic anxiety is often better treated with a course of antidepressant drugs, especially if depression coexists.

Acute severe anxiety can present as an emergency. It may mask a medical problem—such as pain, pulmonary embolism, internal haemorrhage, or drug or alcohol withdrawal—or it may have been provoked by psychological trauma such as seeing another patient die. Whether or not the underlying cause is amenable to specific treatment, sedation is usually required. Lorazepam, a short acting benzodiazepine, can be given as 1 mg or 2.5 mg tablets orally or sublingually, or intravenously as 25-30 µg/kg. Alternatively, midazolam 5-10 mg can be given intravenously or subcutaneously. An antipsychotic such as haloperidol 5-10 mg may be better if the patient is also psychotic or confused. Medical assessment needs to be repeated every few hours, and the continued presence of a skilled and sympathetic companion is helpful.

Some psychological and practical therapies

- Brief psychotherapy—Cognitive-behavioural, cognitive-analytic, problem solving
- Group discussions for information and support
- Music therapy
- Art therapy
- Creative writing
- Relaxation techniques
- Meditation
- Hypnotherapy
- Aromatherapy
- Practical activity—Such as craft work, swimming

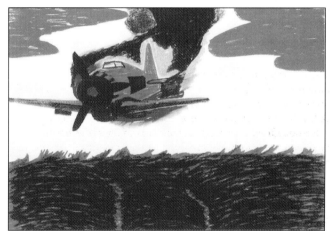

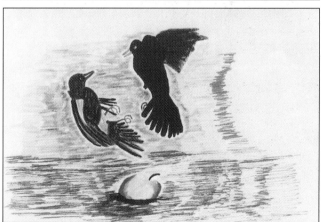

Figure 8.1 Examples of art therapy—The painter of these figures is a man with cancer of the larynx. Having lost his voice, his partner, and his hobby of playing the trumpet, he was depressed, angry, and in pain. He likened himself to an aircraft being shot down in flames or to a frightened bird at the mercy of a larger bird of prey. He has since improved, and wrote to tell his doctor how much it helped to draw his "awful thoughts." (Pictures and case history courtesy of Camilla Connell, art therapist at Royal Marsden Hospital.)

Confusion

It is best to identify any treatable medical causes before prescribing further drugs, which may make the confusion worse. In practice, however, sedation is often required. For mild nocturnal confusion, an antipsychotic such as thioridazine 25-50 mg or haloperidol 1.5-5 mg at bedtime is often sufficient. For severe delirium, a single dose of haloperidol 5-10 mg may be offered in tablet or liquid form or by injection. This may be repeated hourly until a calming effect is achieved, with the dose increasing to 20 mg if necessary. If it does not work a benzodiazepine or a barbiturate can be added.

It may be possible to withdraw the drugs after one or two days if reversible factors such as infection or dehydration have been dealt with. Otherwise, sedation may need to be continued until death, preferably by continuous subcutaneous infusion, for which a suitable regimen might be as much as haloperidol 10-30 mg with midazolam 30-60 mg per 24 hours. These drugs can be mixed in the same syringe.

Outcome

Emotional disorders in patients with incurable disease should never be dismissed as inevitable or untreatable. Worthwhile improvements in psychological state can often be achieved even though the physical illness continues to advance. We must be wary of projecting any sense of hopelessness onto our patients and avoid dismissing anxiety and depression as understandable, thereby denying appropriate treatment in many cases.

"Lifting the heart"
A week ago nothing mattered
I didn't want to do anything
I just wanted to die.
Today something lifted my heart up
Somebody had built some flowers
The newness of new crocuses

These words were written by a man who had been both confused and suicidally depressed after diagnosis of a brain tumour, but whose mental state improved after prescription of amitriptyline. Reproduced from *Throwaway Lines: writing from Sobell House with Lynne Alexander Sobell* Publications, 1991.

9   HIV infection and AIDS

Chris G A Wood, Sally Whittet, Caroline S Bradbeer

When AIDS first emerged as a clinical problem, some 15 years ago, many patients died early from acute illnesses such as pneumocystis carinii pneumonia. Cumulative experience and increased awareness have led to the use of prophylaxis, earlier diagnosis, and more effective treatments for HIV itself and the many complications of HIV infection and AIDS. As a result, patients with AIDS now have improved survival but are more likely to experience months or years of increasing dependency, punctuated by episodes of acute illness.

Currently, the clinical picture is changing through the use of new combinations of antiretroviral drugs, which improve patients' wellbeing and delay disease progression. They are not, however, a cure, and it is likely that they will only delay the disease process for months or a few years at the most. Three drugs are usually used in combination, resulting in problems with drug interactions and compliance.

During the later stages of the disease many patients prefer to remain at home whenever possible, relying on the support of community services. Hospices are then used when residential respite care is needed. In addition, many patients have also been choosing to die at home or in a hospice rather than in hospital. This has meant that increasing numbers of people who are not specialists in HIV infection are needing to become familiar with managing HIV infection, especially in advanced or terminal cases.

Some people with AIDS are very well informed about the illness and may also have experience of caring for partners and friends with AIDS. They can be a valuable source of knowledge for the health workers looking after them. Others are less well informed or are too bewildered and frightened to express their needs clearly. The complexity of the issues involved means that open discussion with patients is needed in order to help establish their medical and personal priorities, and to allow agreement to be reached in balancing realistic therapeutic goals and quality of life.

Natural course of HIV infection

HIV infection has a variable and unpredictable course, with a wide range of potential complications, rates of progression, and survival. Some patients remain free of serious symptoms and complications until they have reached an advanced stage of immunosuppression, while others suffer debilitating malaise and fatigue or frequent non-life threatening complications throughout their infection. Many seem to come to terms with their situation at an early stage, but some find themselves living with daily uncertainty and fear, which may continue for many years. Many also experience a drawn out series of crises relating to emotional, psychological, social, economic, and physical milestones.

People with AIDS are not necessarily ill all of the time and may remain fit and working long after their AIDS defining diagnosis. It is, however, an aging illness, and, as it progresses, patients become increasingly debilitated and dependent on others, ultimately requiring intensive practical support and nursing care. Like elderly people, they may also experience multiple loss through death of peers and family, cognitive impairment, degrees of dementia, reduced mobility, and incontinence. Cachexia and malnourishment are

Cases of AIDS and HIV infection in the United Kingdom*

	Total No of cases		People living with AIDS†
	HIV infection	AIDS	
To end of March 1992	17 494	5782	2152
To end of March 1997	29 107	14 075	2594

*As reported to the Public Health Laboratory Service since 1984
† Calculated by subtracting notified cases

Combination antiretroviral therapy

- Responsible for decrease in death rates, progression to AIDS, inpatient admissions
- Dramatic physical and medical improvement in patients with apparently end stage AIDS
- May help to control previously uncontrollable opportunistic infections and AIDS related symptoms
- Benefits may be time limited, and therapeutic failure is increasingly common
- Complex drug interactions, toxicities, and intolerance
- Requires specialist management

Specific issues in palliative care of AIDS patients

Medical
- Multiple infections
- Chronic suppressive therapy
- Increased risk of adverse drug reactions
- Continued prophylaxis
- Multiple medications

Psychosocial
- Young patients (usually)
- Marginalised or minority groups
- Partners and carers often infected
- Family members often infected
- Often well informed
- Stigmatised
- Confidentiality
- Infected peer networks
- Multiple bereavements
- Fears of "contagion"

Average time from HIV seroconversion to developing AIDS is 8-10 years
Average survival after developing AIDS is 18-30 months

(These times are approximate with considerable variability)

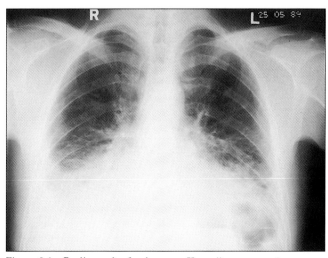

Figure 9.1   Radiograph of pulmonary Kaposi's sarcoma. Average prognosis is 3-9 months

psychologically distressing and increase the risk of developing bedsores. Death is usually due to multiple causes, including chronic incurable systemic infections, malignancies, neurological disease, wasting and malnutrition, and multisystem failure.

Multidisciplinary and shared care

Most people who are infected with HIV obtain their care from a specialist hospital clinic. These clinics usually provide a safe environment and a variety of services, such as access to specialised drugs, walk-in and day care facilities, counselling, complementary treatments, peer support, and advice about services and benefits.

Many patients do not have a general practitioner and are often reluctant to register with one. Even if they are registered they may still not disclose their HIV status. The reasons for this include their concerns over confidentiality, the fear of discrimination, and the risk of rejection because of the belief of potential financial costs to the practice of looking after a patient with AIDS. This means that general practitioners often become involved with AIDS patients only at a late stage in their disease. It is important to encourage patients to register early with a general practitioner in whom they can build trust so that the transition to shared care can be made as smoothly as possible.

It is often feasible to reduce the need for patients with end stage disease to attend hospital by providing care in their homes and using local hospices and services when appropriate. Medical conditions, and thus the required treatments, change frequently in these patients, so good communication between the many agencies involved is essential. This is facilitated by patient held record cards (including updated details of medication) and direct communication by telephone and fax (with care to ensure confidentiality). Named key workers help to coordinate patients' care and also act as patients' advocates if required.

For patients with late disease, prior discussion about advance directives, desired levels of medical intervention in the event of clinical deterioration, and preferred place of death can help to prevent unnecessary hospital visits and inappropriate hospital admissions. Contingency plans need to be made so that patients and carers are clear which agencies should be called in an emergency.

Medical management

Medical management of patients with AIDS is a balance between acute treatment and attempting to control chronic symptoms and conditions. As patients approach the end stage of the illness, they may decline certain investigations and treatments if these seem unlikely to be of much long term benefit.

New symptoms, however, may still warrant invasive investigations because atypical presentations and extensive differential diagnoses can make easily treatable conditions unrecognisable—for example, endoscopy should be considered when investigating retrosternal pain and nausea not responding to antifungal treatment. There are also some distressing symptoms that can be controlled effectively only by specific treatment of the underlying condition (such as perianal infection with herpes simplex virus and oro-oesophageal candida).

While the underlying cause of pain and other symptoms in AIDS is often susceptible to specific treatment, symptomatic treatment should not be delayed. The principles of pain management should follow those outlined in the first article of this series.

Community provision of care for AIDS patients

Individuals
- Informal carers
- General practitioners
- District nurses
- Specialist HIV nurses
- Palliative care nurses
- Community psychiatric nurses
- Social workers
- 'Buddies' (volunteers)
- Community care assistants (including 24 hour cover)
- Community occupational therapists
- Spiritual advisers

Organisations
- Social services
- General hospices
- Specialist HIV hospices
- Local support groups

Contacts for details of services available
- *National AIDS Manual*
  Published yearly
  Telephone (0171) 627 3200
- National AIDS Helpline
  Telephone 0800 567123

Common symptoms in AIDS

Causes	Management
Cough	
Sinus disease with postnasal drip, bacterial chest infection, pneumocystis carinii pneumonia, pulmonary Kaposi's sarcoma, tuberculosis	Sputum for diagnosis, treat specific conditions when appropriate, consider decongestants
Diarrhoea	
Treatable—Salmonella, giardia, campylobacter, clostridium difficile, cytomegalovirus	Stool samples may be appropriate, specific antibacterial treatment
Unresponsive—Cryptosporidium, microsporidium, and 'pathogen negative' diarrhoea	Symptomatic control can be difficult, subcutaneous diamorphine or octreotide may be tried
Anorexia, nausea, vomiting	
Candida, malignancy (early satiety, acute abdomen), drugs, constipation	Review candida treatment, re-evaluate medication, consider antiemetics, dietary advice
Pruritus	
Dry skin, drug reactions, scabies, folliculitis	Emollients, antipruritics, anti-scabies treatment, topical corticosteroids
Malaise, weakness, pyrexia	
May be no detectable cause, drug reactions	Investigate, consider corticosteroids

---

Common causes of pain in AIDS

Oropharyngeal—Candida, herpes viruses (herpes simplex virus, cytomegalovirus, varicella zoster virus), aphthous-type ulcers, malignancy, gingivitis, tooth abscesses
Retrosternal—Oesophageal candida, infection with cytomegalovirus or herpes simplex virus, giant oesophageal ulcers, reflux oesophagitis, pneumocystis carinii pneumonia
Headache—Toxoplasmosis, cryptococcal meningitis, cerebral lymphoma
Abdominal—Diarrhoea with or without infection, AIDS related sclerosing cholangitis, malignancy (such as Kaposi's sarcoma, lymphoma), drugs (such as clarithromycin), constipation
Perianal and perineal—Herpes simplex virus (very common, needs high index of suspicion), candida, excoriation of skin due to diarrhoea

Patients entering the terminal phases of disease are often receiving several drugs because many symptoms and conditions need continued prophylaxis or chronic suppressive treatment. Uncontrolled cytomegalovirus retinitis, for example, can cause blindness, so usually needs to be actively managed until death. Systemic infection with mycobacterium avium complex, may cause general malaise with fevers, anaemia, and debilitating fatigue. In this situation specific treatment of the infection, which usually involves two or three drugs, may be appropriate, or use of corticosteroids for further palliation of symptoms may be considered.

Drug treatments should be reviewed regularly so that clinical problems are controlled with a minimum of polypharmacy. Patients with AIDS and clinical or subclinical dementia can be susceptible to cognitive impairment with various drugs—sedatives, anxiolytics, strong opioids, and antidepressants.

Management of nutritional and dietary intake is also important for both medical and psychological reasons. In the final stages of AIDS, combination antiretroviral treatment may be helpful, but it is less effective than earlier in the disease and decisions about continuation should be taken with the patient.

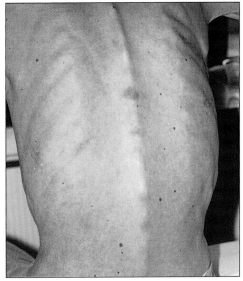

Figure 9.2 Wasting is common in Aids and can cause pain, bed sores, and psychological distress

Common conditions in AIDS that require active management until death

	Presentation and symptoms	Treatment
Cytomegalovirus retinitis	Potential blindness, scotomas	Intravenous ganciclovir, foscarnet (needs indwelling catheter such as PortaCath or Hickman line); oral ganciclovir may be appropriate in some cases. These drugs are expensive and must be prescribed by hospital doctor
Candidiasis	*Oropharyngeal or oesophageal*—Painful oropharynx, retrosternal pain, dysphagia, anorexia, nausea and vomiting. Even mild oral candidiasis can be symptomatic and associated with oesophageal candida	Fluconazole or itraconazole (may need up to four times recommended dose as resistance common in advanced AIDS). Intravenous amphotericin (intermittent treatment may be needed in resistant cases)
Herpes simplex virus	*Oropharyngeal or anogenital*—Pain, paraesthesia, ulcers. Patients may complain of 'piles' or bleeding from rectum	Aciclovir for acute episode (may need maintenance and up to four times recommended dose)
Mycobacterium avium complex	Fevers, night sweats, malaise, fatigue, anorexia, weight loss, diarrhoea, anaemia; symptoms may occur singly or in combination	Combination therapy (such as rifabutin, clarithromycin, and ethambutol) may give good palliation of symptoms. Single drug for short periods if compliance or polypharmacy a problem
Kaposi's sarcoma	*Pulmonary*—Cough, dry or productive and may be paroxysms; progressive breathlessness; haemoptysis; effusions	Symptomatic control (such as anxiolytics, opioids, oxygen). Chemotherapy and radiotherapy of limited value. Poor prognosis
	Cutaneous, lymphatic, or other viscera—Local symptoms such as lymphadenopathy, oedema, loss of function, breakdown or necrosis of skin, pain, possible severe disfigurement and distortion of tissues	Variable natural course (minor or considerable morbidity). Chemotherapy and radiotherapy may help palliation of problems. Corticosteroids can help oedema but may exacerbate infections
AIDS dementia complex	Variable neurological presentations, including dementia and psychiatric illness	Difficult and distressing to manage, requiring multidisciplinary approach. Combination therapy, which must include high dose zidovudine, is worth trying
Pneumocystis carinii pneumonia	Dry cough, possibly paroxysmal and distressing; chest pain; breathlessness; fevers; sweats; malaise; anorexia	Prophylaxis (primary or secondary) usually continued (co-trimoxazole, dapsone, pentamidine)
Co-infection with hepatitis B or C	Usually incidental finding with liver function tests	Poor response to treatment. Complicates prescribing of hepatotoxic drugs

Social and cultural issues

Many of those affected by HIV infection and AIDS belong to marginalised or stigmatised minority groups. Management of psychosocial problems may come to dominate the provision of palliative and terminal care. Carers also need adequate support, as many of them may be infected and facing, or already living with, AIDS themselves. Financial help (including advice on benefits, disability allowances, and other support) should be discussed and reviewed regularly.

AIDS related problems with body image

- Wasting
- Severe facial dermatitis
- Permanent indwelling line
- Weakness and dependency
- Slowing of mental functions
- Loss of libido
- Premature greying and loss of hair
- Facial molluscum contagiosum
- Kaposi's sarcoma—common on face
- Progressive visual loss from retinitis
- Incontinence (especially faecal)

Patients and families may express concern about "AIDS" being written on the death certificate, and discussion of this issue can be helpful. Many doctors write a non-specific diagnosis on the main certificate and sign section B on the reverse side (this signifies to the Registrar General that further information will be available later). Doctors should supply voluntary confidential notification of deaths to the Communicable Disease Surveillance Centre (CDSC).

Homosexual men may not have disclosed their sexual orientation, and families may not learn of their illness until it is advanced. Conflicts can arise between a patient's family and partner as to who is the main carer. Homosexual partnerships are not recognised legally in Britain, so patients should make an unambiguous will and specify their preferred "next of kin" or executor.

Immigrant groups—Most patients are from Africa, and in some immigrant communities the stigma of HIV infection is so severe that patients may avoid disclosing their HIV status to almost anyone. This can lead to reduced uptake of services that are identifiably HIV related (such as AIDS hospices and "AIDS wards"). Reassurance about confidentiality and the option of "discreet" services may be useful. Uncertain immigration status can cause great anxiety and can also prevent family members from entering Britain to visit or care for their dying relative.

Haemophiliacs—There are specific medical problems relating to haemophilia (including liver disease due to chronic infection with hepatitis B and C). More than one brother may be affected, and issues of parental guilt and multiple bereavement may arise.

Misusers of injected drugs—Management may be complicated by drug misuse. Ideally, patients should be managed in collaboration with a drug dependency unit, which should take primary responsibility for prescribing opioid maintenance therapy. Many doctors are reluctant to prescribe opioid analgesia to known drug misusers. A patient's pain should be properly assessed and, if necessary, the opioid dose adjusted in relation to the habitual opioid intake. An adequate dose to control pain will often abolish drug seeking behaviour.

Children and families—When both parents are sick, child care or fostering may be needed urgently. Care plans should be made well in advance for any children (whether infected or not) who are likely to be orphaned. Some infected parents fear that their children will be taken into care, and they may conceal their own diagnosis or deny the existence of their children to the authorities or health workers. Parents need help to discuss HIV, AIDS, and death with their children. Management of infected children needs collaboration with a specialist paediatric unit.

Conclusion

Looking after patients with AIDS can seem daunting. It affects young people who are often assertive and well informed, and there may be complex psychosocial issues. The variety of potential medical problems requires multiple medications (some needing an indwelling intravenous catheter) and diagnostic vigilance right up until the end.

Some people with AIDS never come to terms with their illness and impending death, although effective palliative care and management of their special needs can help to avoid unnecessary suffering and provide comfort for them and their bereaved families. It can also enable patients to take control at the end of their lives, allowing them to choose the place of death in the environment and company of their choice. Patients and their carers often display remarkable courage and fortitude, and, despite the inevitable tragedy, a satisfactory death can be a rewarding experience for those involved in their care.

Legal issues
- "Living wills," advance directives
- "Next of kin," executors
- Wills—especially important when partner is not the legal spouse, as in homosexual relationships
- Immigration status
- Death certificates
- Guardianship and provision for orphaned children

Social and cultural issues
Homosexual men
- Sexual orientation may not have been disclosed to families
- Conflicts between patient's partner and family about caring roles and inheritance

Haemophiliacs
- Issues of parental guilt and blame for administering infected clotting factors
- Multiple loss within families

Misusers of injected drugs
- Problems of continuing drug misuse
- Non-conformist behaviour
- Chaotic lifestyles affecting compliance with treatment

Immigrant groups
- Isolation, especially from extended family
- Fear of stigmatisation within cultural community in Britain and for families in country of origin
- Issues of language and cross cultural communication—These can be avoided by using an agency that provides culturally appropriate advice and interpreters
- Past trauma in country of origin

Children and families
- More than one family member may be infected
- Issues of child care and provision for orphans
- Fear of social services "taking children away"
- Care of a dying child

Control of infection
- Extremely low risk of infection to health workers and household contacts
- HIV present in blood and bodily fluids—Gloves to be worn when risk of direct contact with these fluids
- Main risk is direct parenteral inoculation of bodily fluids—Can be reduced by immediate use of antiretroviral drugs
- No risk from casual household contact—Gloves not necessary for normal examination or contact
- Spillages (blood, faeces, urine)—Use ordinary household bleach
- Cutlery, linen, bath, etc—All can be cleaned with ordinary washing products

10 Emergencies

Stephen Falk, Marie Fallon

The concept of rapid assessment, evaluation, and management of symptoms due to malignancy is generally accepted. Inherent in this concept is rapid reversal of what is reversible. Some acute events in malignancy have to be treated as an emergency if a favourable outcome is to be achieved. As in any emergency, the assessment must be as prompt and complete as possible. In patients with advanced malignancy, factors to consider include

- The nature of the emergency
- The general physical condition of the patient
- Disease status and likely prognosis
- Concomitant pathologies
- Symptomatology
- The likely effectiveness and toxicity of available treatments
- Patients' and carers' wishes.

While unnecessary hospital admission may cause distress for the patient and carers, missed emergency treatment of reversible symptomatology can be disastrous.

Hypercalcaemia

Hypercalcaemia is the commonest life threatening metabolic disorder encountered in patients with cancer. The incidence varies with the underlying malignancy, being most common in multiple myeloma and breast cancer (40-50%), less so in non-small cell lung cancer, and rare in small cell lung cancer and colorectal cancer.

It is important to remember non-malignant causes of hypercalcaemia—particularly primary hyperparathyroidism, which is prevalent in the general population.

The pathology of hypercalcaemia is mediated by factors such as parathyroid related protein, prostaglandins, and local interaction by cytokines such as interleukin 1 and tumour necrosis factor. Bone metastases are commonly but not invariably present.

Management

Mild hypercalcaemia (corrected serum calcium concentration ≤ 3.00 mmol/l) is usually asymptomatic, and treatment is required only if a patient has symptoms. For more severe hypercalcaemia, however, treatment can markedly improve symptoms even when a patient has the advanced disease and limited life expectancy to make the end stages less traumatic for patient and carers.

Treatment with bisphosphonate normalises the serum calcium concentration in 80% of patients within a week. Treatment with calcitonin or mithramycin is now largely obsolete. Corticosteroids are probably useful only when the underlying tumour is responsive to this cytostatic agent—such as myeloma, lymphoma, and some carcinomas of the breast.

Some symptoms, particularly confusion, may be slow to improve after treatment despite normalisation of the serum calcium. Always consider treating the underlying malignancy to prevent recurrence of symptoms, since the median duration of normocalcaemia after bisphosphonate infusion is only three weeks. However, if effective systemic therapy has been exhausted, or is deemed inappropriate, oral bisphosphonates (such as clodronate 800 mg twice daily) or parenteral infusions (every three to four weeks) should be considered.

Major emergencies in palliative care

- Hypercalcaemia
- Superior venal caval obstruction
- Spinal cord compression
- Bone fractures

Other emergencies, such as haemorrhage and acute anxiety and depression, are discussed elsewhere in this series

---

Questions to ask when considering management of emergencies in patients with advanced disease

- What is the problem?
- Can it be reversed?
- What effect will reversal of the symptom have on a patient's overall condition?
- What is your medical judgment?
- What does the patient want?
- What do the carers want?
- Could active treatment maintain or improve this patient's quality of life?

Presenting features of hypercalcaemia

Mild symptoms
- Nausea
- Anorexia and vomiting
- Constipation
- Thirst and polyuria

Severe symptoms and signs
- Gross dehydration
- Drowsiness
- Confusion and coma
- Abnormal neurology
- Cardiac arrhythmias

Management of hypercalcaemia

1. Check serum concentration of urea, electrolytes, albumin, and calcium
2. Calculate corrected calcium concentration
- Corrected Ca = measured Ca + (40−albumin)×0.02 mmol/l
- Corrected calcium value is used for treatment decisions

3. Rehydrate with intravenous fluid (0.9% saline)
- Amount and rate depends on clinical and cardiovascular status and concentrations of urea and electrolytes

4. After minimum of 2 l of intravenous fluids give bisphosphonate infusion
- Disodium pamidronate (60 mg if corrected Ca < 3.5 mmol/l, 90 mg if corrected Ca ≥ 3.5 mmol/l) over 2 hours *or*
- Sodium clodronate 1500 mg over 4 hours
- Both given in 0.5 litre 0.9% saline

5. Measure concentrations of urea and electrolytes at daily intervals and give intravenous fluids as necessary
- Normalisation of serum calcium takes 3-5 days
- Do not measure serum calcium for at least 48 hours after rehydration as it may rise transiently immediately after treatment

6. Prevent recurrence of symptoms
- Treat underlying malignancy if possible *or*
- Consider maintenance treatment with bisphosphonates and monitor serum calcium at 3 week intervals *or*
- Monitor serum calcium at 3 week intervals, or less if patient symptomatic, and repeat bisphosphonate infusion as appropriate

Maintenance intravenous bisphosphonates may be administered at a day centre or outpatient department. Oral preparations have the disadvantages of being poorly absorbed and have to be taken at least one hour before or after food. The evidence for intravenous or oral bisphosphonates in preventing recurrence is equal, and choice depends on the individual.

Superior venal caval obstruction

This may arise from occlusion by extrinsic pressure, intraluminal thrombosis, or direct invasion of the vessel wall. Most cases are due to tumour within the mediastinum, of which up to 75% will be primary bronchial carcinomas. About 3% of patients with carcinoma of the bronchus and 8% of those with lymphoma will develop superior venal caval obstruction.

Management

Conventionally, superior venal caval obstruction has been regarded as an oncological emergency requiring immediate treatment. If it is the first presentation of malignancy, treatment will be tempered by the need to obtain an accurate histological diagnosis in order to tailor treatment for potentially curable diseases, such as lymphomas or germ cell tumours, and for diseases such as small cell lung cancer that are better treated with chemotherapy at presentation.

In advanced disease, patients need relief of acute symptoms—of which dyspnoea and a sensation of drowning can be most frightening—and high dose corticosteroids and radiotherapy should be considered. In non-small cell lung cancer palliative radiotherapy gives symptomatic improvement in 70% of patients, with a median duration of palliation of three months. Up to 17% of patients may survive for a year. If radiotherapy is contraindicated or being awaited corticosteroids alone (dexamethasone 16 mg/day) may give relief. In those for whom further radiotherapy is not indicated, stenting (with or without thrombolysis) of the superior vena cava should be considered.

Urgent initiation of pharmacological, practical, and psychological management of dyspnoea is paramount and usually includes opioids, with or without benzodiazepines. Opioid doses are usually small—such as 5 mg morphine every 4 hours. It is important to review all corticosteroid prescriptions in view of their potential adverse effects. We recommend stopping corticosteroids after five days if no benefit is obtained, and a gradual reduction in dose for those who have responded.

Spinal cord compression

> **Presentation of spinal cord compression can be very subtle in the early stages. Any patient with back pain and subtle neurological symptoms or signs should have radiological investigations, with magnetic resonance imaging when possible**

This occurs in up to 5% of cancer patients. The main problem in clinical practice is failure of recognition. It is not uncommon for patients' weak legs to be attributed to general debility, and urinary and bowel symptoms to be attributed to medication. Neurological symptoms and signs can vary from subtle to gross, from upper motor neurone to lower motor neurone, and from minor sensory changes to clearly demarcated sensory loss.

Prompt treatment is essential if function is to be maintained: neurological status at the start of treatment is the most important factor influencing outcome. If treatment is started within 24-48 hours of onset of symptoms neurological damage may be reversible.

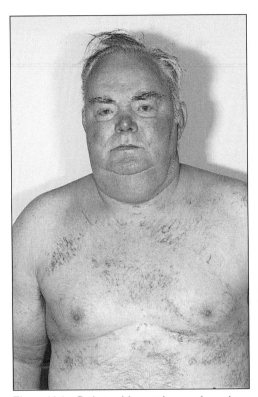

Figure 10.1 Patient with superior venal caval obstruction showing typical signs (reproduced with patient's permission)

Spinal cord compression can arise from intradural metastasis but is more commonly extradural in origin. In 85% of cases cord damage arises from extension of a vertebral body metastasis into the epidural space, but other mechanisms of damage include vertebral collapse, direct spread of tumour through the intervertebral foramen (usually in lymphoma or testicular tumour), and interruption of the vascular supply.

The frequency with which a spinal level is affected reflects the number and volume of vertebral bodies in each segment—about 10% of compressions are cervical, 70% thoracic, and 20% lumbosacral. It is important to remember that more than one site of compression may occur, and this is increasingly recognised with improved imaging techniques.

The earliest symptom of spinal cord compression is back pain, sometimes with symptoms of root irritation, causing a girdle-like pain, often described as a "band," that tends to be worse on coughing or straining. Most patients have pain for weeks or months before they start to detect weakness. Initially, stiffness rather than weakness may be a feature, and tingling and numbness usually starts in both feet and ascends the legs. In contrast to pain, the start of myelopathy is usually rapid. Urinary symptoms such as hesitancy or incontinence and perianal numbness are late features. Increasing compression of the spinal cord is often marked by improvement or resolution of the back pain but can be associated with worsening of pain.

Examination may reveal a demarcated area of sensory loss and brisk or absent reflexes, which may help to localise the lesion. In patients unfit to undergo more detailed investigations, plain radiology can reveal erosion of the pedicles, vertebral collapse, and, occasionally, a large paravertebral mass. These may help in the application of palliative radiotherapy. In contrast to myelography with localised computed tomographic *x* rays for soft tissue detail, magnetic resonance imaging is now considered the investigation of choice: it is non-invasive and shows the whole spine, enabling detection of multiple areas of compression.

Management

> **Decisions on investigations performed and treatment given will depend on the patient's wishes and the stage of the disease. Only in exceptional circumstances will corticosteroids not form part of the treatment plan**

After palliative radiotherapy, 70% of patients who were ambulatory at the start of treatment retain their ability to walk and 35% of paraparetic patients regain their ability to walk, while only 5% of completely paraplegic patients do so. These figures underline the importance of early diagnosis, since 75% of patients have substantial weakness at presentation to oncology units.

Retrospective analysis has not shown an advantage for patients managed by laminectomy and radiotherapy over radiotherapy alone. Surgical decompression is therefore now performed less routinely and is usually reserved for cases when

- A tissue diagnosis is required (if biopsy guided by computed tomography is not possible)
- Deterioration occurs during radiotherapy
- There is bone destruction causing spinal cord compression.

For a small number of fit patients with disease anterior to the spinal canal, excellent results have been reported for an anterior approach for surgical decompression and vertebral stabilisation—80% of the patients became ambulant. For relief of the mechanical problems due to bone collapse, laminectomy decompression has to be accompanied by spinal stabilisation. Such surgery is difficult and not always appropriate.

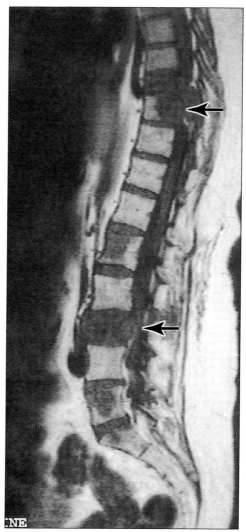

Figure 10.2   Magnetic resonance image showing patient with spinal cord compression at two different sites (arrows)

Management of spinal cord compression

Main points
- Except for unusual circumstances give oral dexamethasone 16 mg/day
- Urgent treatment, definitely within 24 hours of start of symptoms
- Interdisciplinary approach involving oncologists, neurosurgeons, radiologists, nurses, physiotherapists, occupational therapists

Treatment options
- Continue with dexamethasone 16 mg/day *plus*
- Radiation only
   For most situations
   Radiosensitive tumour without spinal instability
- Surgery and radiation
   Spinal instability, such as fracture or compression by bone
   No tissue diagnosis (when needle biopsy guided by computed tomography not possible)
- Surgery only
   Relapse at previously irradiated area
   Progression during radiotherapy
- Chemotherapy
   Paediatric tumours responsive to chemotherapy
   Adjuvant treatment for adult tumours responsive to chemotherapy
   Relapse of previously irradiated tumour responsive to chemotherapy
- Corticosteroids alone
   Final stages of terminal illness and patient either too unwell to have radiotherapy or unlikely to live long enough to have any benefits

Bone fracture

Bone metastases are a common feature of advanced cancer. Bone fracture may also be due to osteoporosis or trauma. Fractures can present in a variety of forms, including as an acute confusional state.

Management

If fracture of a long bone seems likely, as judged by the presence of cortical thinning, prophylactic internal fixation should be considered. Once a fracture has occurred the available options include external or internal fixation—their relative merits are determined by the site of the fracture and the general condition of the patient.

Radiotherapy is usually given in an attempt to enhance healing and to prevent further progression of the bony metastasis and subsequent loosening of any fixation.

Evidence exists that, when combined with oncolytic therapy in breast cancer and multiple myeloma, oral bisphosphonates can reduce skeletal morbidity (hypercalcaemia, vertebral fracture, and need for palliative radiotherapy).

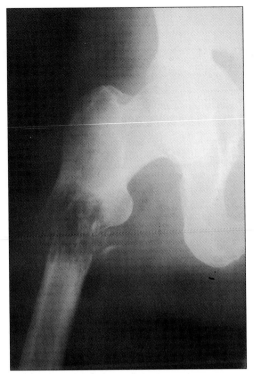

Figure 10.3   Radiograph showing pathological fracture of the femur

11   The last 48 hours

Jim Adam

During the final 48 hours of life, patients experience increasing weakness and immobility, loss of interest in food and drink, difficulty swallowing, and drowsiness. With an incurable and progressive illness, this phase can usually be anticipated, but sometimes a deterioration can be sudden and distressing. Control of symptoms and family support take priority, and the nature of the primary illness becomes less important. This is a time when levels of anxiety, stress, and emotion can be high for patients, families, and other carers. It is important that the healthcare team adopts a sensitive yet structured approach.

Principles

An analytical approach to symptom control continues but usually relies on clinical findings rather than investigation. This approach spans all causes of terminal illness and applies to care at home, hospital, or hospice.

Drugs are reviewed with regard to need and route of administration. Previously "essential" drugs such as antihypertensives, corticosteroids, antidepressants, and hypoglycaemics are often no longer needed and analgesic, antiemetic, sedative, and anticonvulsant drugs form the new "essential" list to work from. The route of administration depends on the clinical situation and characteristics of the drugs used. Some patients manage to take oral drugs until near to death, but many require an alternative route. Any change in medication relies on information from patient, family, and carers (both lay and professional) and regular medical review to monitor the level of symptom control and side effects.

This review should include an assessment of how the family and carers are coping; effective communication with all involved should be maintained and lines of communication made clear and open. The knowledge that help is available is often a reassurance and can influence the place of death.

Symptom control

Pain

Pain control is achievable in 80% of patients by following the World Health Organisation's guidelines for use of analgesic drugs, as outlined in the first chapter of this series. A patient's history and examination are used to assess all likely causes of pain, both benign and malignant. Treatment (usually with an opioid) is individually tailored, the effect reviewed, and dose titrated accordingly. Acute episodes of pain are dealt with urgently in the same analytical fashion but require more frequent review and provision of appropriate "breakthrough" analgesia. If a patient is already receiving analgesia then this is continued through the final stages; pain may disturb an unconscious patient since the original cause of the pain still exists.

If oral administration is no longer possible the subcutaneous route provides a simple and effective alternative. Diamorphine is the strong opioid of choice because of its solubility and is delivered through a infusion device to avoid repeated injections every four hours. It can be mixed with other "essential" drugs in the syringe driver. Rectal administration is another alternative, but the need for suppositories every four hours in

---

Principles of managing the last 48 hours

- Problem solving approach to symptom control
- Avoid unnecessary interventions
- Review all drugs and symptoms regularly
- Maintain effective communication
- Ensure support for family and carers

Routes of administration of drugs for last 48 hours

Oral
All drug types

Sublingual

Antiemetic	Hyoscine hydrobromide 0.3 mg/6 hours (Kwells) Prochlorperazine 3-6 mg/12 hours
Sedative or anxiolytic	Lorazepam 0.5-2 mg/6 hours (fast acting and short duration)

Transdermal

Opioid	Fentanyl (only if patient already using patches)
Antiemetic	Hyoscine hydrobromide 0.5 mg/72 hours (Transcop)

Subcutaneous*

Opioid	Diamorphine (individual dose titration)
Non-steroidal anti-inflammatory drug	Diclofenac (infusion) 150 mg/24 hours
Antiemetics	Cyclizine† 25-50 mg bolus every 8 hours, up to 150 mg/24 hours Metoclopramide‡ 10 mg bolus every 6 hours, 40-80 mg/24 hours Hyoscine hydrobromide‡ (also dries secretions) 0.4-0.6 mg bolus, up to 2.4 mg/24 hours Methotrimeprazine‡ (also sedative at higher doses) 25 mg/ml ampoule, 6.25-25 mg bolus, 6.25 mg titrated up to 250 mg/24 hours via syringe driver
Sedatives	Haloperidol‡ (also useful for confusion with altered sensorium) 2.5-5 mg bolus, 5-20 mg/24 hours Midazolam‡ (anxiolytic at smaller doses, anticonvulsant) 2.5-10 mg bolus, 5-60 mg/24 hours
Somatostatin analogue	Octreotide‡ (for large volume vomit associated with bowel obstruction) 150-600 µg/24 hours

---

Rectal

Opioid	Morphine (individual dose made by pharmacist taken every 4 hours) Oxycodone 30-60 mg/8 hours
Non-steroidal anti-inflammatory drug	Diclofenac 100 mg once daily
Antiemetic	Prochlorperazine 25 mg twice daily Domperidone 30-60 mg/6 hours Cyclizine 50 mg/8 hours Chlorpromazine (also sedative) 100 mg/8 hours (equivalent to 50 mg/8 hours orally)
Sedative	Diazepam (also anxiolytic and anticonvulsant) rectal tubes 5-10 mg

*All subcutaneous preparations diluted in sterile water except diclofenac (0.9% saline)
†Compatible with diamorphine but liable to precipitate as concentrations increase
‡Compatible with diamorphine

the case of morphine limits its usefulness. Oxycodone suppositories (repeated 8 hourly) may be more practicable.

Longer acting opioid preparations (transdermal fentanyl and sustained release morphine) should not be started in a patient close to death; there is a variable delay in reaching effective levels, and, since speedy dose titration is difficult, they are unsuitable for situations where a rapid effect is required, such as uncontrolled pain. If a patient is already prescribed fentanyl patches these should be continued as baseline analgesia; if pain escalates additional quick acting analgesia (immediate release morphine or diamorphine) should be titrated against the pain.

Not all pains are best dealt with by opioids. For example, bone pain may be helped by a non-steroidal anti-inflammatory drug, while muscle spasm may be eased by diazepam. Non-drug measures still apply: for example, pain from a dry mouth requires mouth care; a pressure sore requires a change of position, a comfort dressing, local anaesthetic gel, and an appropriate mattress; and a distended bladder and loaded rectum require catheterisation and rectal evacuation respectively. It is also important to remember all the non-cancer pains, new and old, that may be present.

Breathlessness

The scope for correcting "reversible" causes of breathlessness becomes limited. A notable exception is cardiac failure, for which diuresis may be effective. In most cases the priority is to address the symptom of breathlessness and the fear and anxiety that may accompany it.

General supportive measures should be considered in all cases. Face masks may be uncomfortable or intrusive at this time, but oxygen therapy may help some patients (even in the absence of hypoxia). Nebulised 0.9% saline is useful if a patient has a dry cough or sticky secretions but should be avoided if bronchospasm is present.

Opioids and benzodiazepines can be helpful and should be initiated at low doses. Immediate release morphine can be titrated to effect in the same way as for pain. If a patient is using morphine for pain control then a dose slightly higher than the appropriate breakthrough dose (oral or parenteral) is usually required for treating acute breathlessness. The choice of anxiolytic is often determined by what is the most suitable route of administration, but the speed and duration of action are important.

Noisy respiration may be helped by repositioning the patient and, if substantial secretions are present, hyoscine hydrobromide (0.4-0.6 mg subcutaneous bolus or up to 2.4 mg/ 24 hours via infusion device). Occasionally, gentle suction may be required. End stage stridor is managed with opioids and anxiolytics, when it is usually too late for corticosteroids.

Restlessness and confusion

These may be distinct entities or they may overlap. A problem solving approach is essential. The threshold for discomfort and disorientation is often lowered in cachectic or anxious patients. Attention to a patient's surroundings is therefore important—a stable, comfortable, and safe environment should be fostered; soft light, quiet, and familiar faces are reassuring.

The key to treatment lies in calming the acute state while addressing the cause, if apparent and appropriate. A notable example is the mental clouding, hallucinations, confusion, and restlessness associated with opioid toxicity, which can be eased with haloperidol while the opioid dose is reviewed. In general, choice of drug treatment depends on the likely cause. Doses are titrated up or down to achieve the desired effect, and the situation should be reviewed regularly and often until the acute

---

Opioid treatment for pain control

Starting dose—Immediate release morphine 5 mg every 4 hours by mouth

Increments—A third of current dose (but varies according to 'breakthrough analgesia' required in previous 24 hours). For example, immediate release morphine 15 mg every 4 hours by mouth is increased to 20 mg/4 hours

Breakthrough analgesia—A sixth of 24 hour dose. For example, with diamorphine 60 mg delivered subcutaneously by syringe driver over 24 hours, give diamorphine 10 mg subcutaneously as needed for breakthrough pain

Conversion ratio—Morphine by mouth (or rectum) to subcutaneous diamorphine is 3:1. For example, sustained release morphine 30 mg every 12 hours by mouth plus three doses of immediate release morphine 10 mg by mouth gives total dose of oral morphine 90 mg every 24 hours; convert to diamorphine 30 mg/24 hours delivered subcutaneously

---

Management of breathlessness

- Reverse what is reversible
- General supportive measures—Explanation, position, breathing exercises, fan or cool airflow, relaxation techniques
- Oxygen therapy
- Opioid
- Benzodiazepine
- Hyoscine
- Nebulised saline (if no bronchospasm and patient able to expectorate)

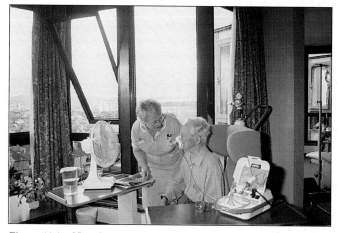

Figure 11.1   Non-drug measures which can help a breathless patient

---

Causes of restlessness and confusion

- Drugs—Such as opioids, corticosteroids, neuroleptics, alcohol (intoxication and withdrawal)
- Physical—Unrelieved pain, distended bladder or bowel, immobility or exhaustion, cerebral lesions, infection, haematological abnormalities, major organ failure
- Metabolic upset—Urea, calcium, sodium, glucose, hypoxia
- Anxiety and distress

episode settles. Highly agitated patients may need a large dose, and continuous infusion may be needed. Rectally administered drugs are possible alternatives. Explanation and support for the relatives and carers are paramount at this time.

If a patient is experiencing distressing twitching or jerks then metabolic disorders, opioid toxicity, or drugs that lower seizure threshold should be considered. A review of medication and treatment with a benzodiazepine or anticonvulsant (such as clonazepam orally, diazepam rectally, or midazolam subcutaneously) is indicated. Anxiety or distress not responding to general supportive measures may be helped by diazepam or midazolam, but it should always be remembered that a patient may be suffering from an emotional or spiritual anguish that cannot be relieved by drugs.

Nausea and vomiting

If antiemetics have been needed within the previous 24 hours then continuation is advisable. Nausea and vomiting may rarely occur as a new symptom at this time (< 10% of cases), and treatment of the likely cause is preferred if this is practical in the clinical situation, otherwise an appropriate antiemetic should be selected. If the aetiology is unclear then choose a centrally acting or broad spectrum antiemetic in the first instance.

Occasionally, more than one antiemetic is required if resistant vomiting of a multifactorial cause exists. Subcutaneous administration of antiemetics is preferable, but suppositories (such as prochlorperazine, cyclizine, or domperidone) may be useful if subcutaneous infusion is not possible. Antiemetic treatment that has been initiated for bowel obstruction should be continued.

Emergency situations

Appropriate and timely action has an important immediate effect on patients and families. It can also influence bereavement and future coping mechanisms of both lay and professional carers. Emergencies can sometimes be anticipated: thus, previous haemoptysis may predict haemorrhage, bone metastases predict pathological fracture, enlarging upper airway tumour predict stridor, and previous hypercalcaemia predict confusion.

Some emergencies may be preventable. For example, a patient with a brain tumour who can no longer take corticosteroids may have a seizure unless anticonvulsant treatment is maintained: subcutaneous infusion of midazolam (starting at 30 mg/24 hours) and rectally administered diazepam (10 mg) may be the strategy required.

However, most emergencies in the last 48 hours are irreversible, and treatment should be aimed at the urgent relief of distress and concomitant symptoms. Drugs should be made available for immediate administration by nursing staff without further consultation with a doctor. Directions regarding use should be written clearly in unambiguous language. Useful drugs are injections of midazolam (5-10 mg if patient not previously exposed to benzodiazepine, otherwise titrate as appropriate) and diamorphine (5-10 mg if no prior exposure to opioid, otherwise a sixth to a third of the 24 hour dose).

Haemorrhage is distressing and memorable for both patients and carers. Haemoptysis, haematemesis, and erosion of a major artery such as the carotid are visually traumatic. The prompt use of drugs, dark coloured towels to make the view less distressing (green surgical towels in hospital), and warmth will aid comfort. In these situations death may occur quickly. A supportive presence is helpful, and explanations to patients and their carers of what is being done will help minimise distress in a crisis.

Management of restlessness and confusion

- Treat the acute state and address cause
- General supportive measures—Light, reassurance, company
- Choice of drug treatment relates to likely cause

Drugs
- Haloperidol
  Indications—Drug toxicity, altered sensorium, metabolic upset
  Dose—Oral drug 1.5-3 mg, repeat after 1 hour and review; subcutaneous bolus 2.5-10 mg; subcutaneous infusion 5-30 mg over 24 hours
- Midazolam
  Indications—Anxiety and distress, risk of seizure
  Dose—Subcutaneous bolus 2.5-10 mg; subcutaneous infusion 5-100 mg over 24 hours
- Methotrimeprazine
  Indications—Need for alternative or additional sedation
  Dose—Subcutaneous bolus 25 mg; subcutaneous infusion up to 250 mg over 24 hours (lowers seizure threshold, use with care)
- For altered sensorium plus anxiety, combine haloperidol and midazolam
- Avoid 'slippery slope' of inappropriate sedation in patient who needs to talk—So called "terminal agitation" can result from the inappropriate use of drugs

---

Causes and treatment of nausea and vomiting

Site of effect	Treatment
Drugs or biochemical upset Chemoreceptor trigger zone (area postrema) via dopamine receptors	Haloperidol
Raised intracranial pressure Vomiting centre(s) via histamine receptors	Cyclizine
Multifactorial or uncertain Various	Methotrimeprazine
Gastrointestinal stasis Gastrokinetic	Metoclopramide Cisapride
Bowel obstruction Vomiting centre(s) via vagus nerve Gastrointestinal secretions	Cyclizine Octreotide Hyoscine butylbromide

---

Emergencies

- Stridor
- Seizure
- Haemorrhage
- Pain
- Confusion

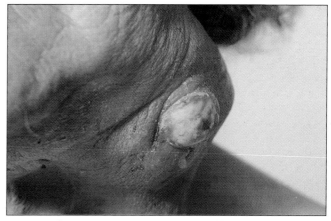

Figure 11.2 Patient with ulcerated neck tumour at risk of erosion of the carotid artery and massive bleed

Support

Support means recognising and addressing the physical and emotional issues that may face patients, families, and carers during this time. Honesty, listening, availability, and assurance that symptom control will continue are valued by patients and carers. Fears or religious concerns should be acknowledged and addressed appropriately, and respect for cultural differences should be assured. Explain what is happening, what is likely to happen, the drugs being used, the support available, and how the family can help with care.

Lack of practical support is one of the commonest reasons for admission to hospital or hospice at this time, and, therefore, consideration should be given to extra help—such as Marie Curie nurses (organised through the district nursing service) to give carers rest and support. An assessment of the risk of bereavement allows care to be planned for the family after the patient's death. Professional carers may also need support, particularly if the last 48 hours have been difficult, and this requires an open line of communication.

Risk factors for bereavement

Patient—young
Illness—Short, protracted, disfiguring, distressing
Death—Sudden, traumatic (such as haemorrhage)
Relationship—Ambivalent, hostile, dependent
Main carer—Young, other dependants, physical or mental illness, concurrent crises, little or no support

---

12 Special problems of children

Ann Goldman

The death of a child has long been acknowledged as one of the greatest tragedies that can happen to a family, and care for seriously ill children and their families is central to paediatrics. It is only recently, however, that the needs for palliative care of children with life limiting illnesses and their families have been considered as a speciality within paediatrics: the most suitable approaches to care are still being developed, and the provision of services nationally is uneven and sometimes inadequate.

Which children need care?

Fortunately, deaths in childhood that can be anticipated, and for which palliative care can be planned, are rare. A recent joint report by ACT (Association for Children with Life Threatening or Terminal Conditions and their Families) and the Royal College of Paediatrics and Child Health offers the most up to date information about epidemiology (see box of further reading).

Paediatric palliative care may be needed for a wide range of diseases, which differ from adult diseases and many of which are rare and familial. The diagnosis influences the type of care that a child and family will need, and four broad groups have been identified.

Palliative care may be needed from infancy and for many years for some children, while others may not need it until they are older and only for a short time. Also the transition between aggressive treatments to cure or prolong good quality life and palliative care may not be clear—both approaches may be needed in conjunction, each becoming dominant at different times.

Aspects of care in children

Child development

An intrinsic aspect of childhood is children's continuing physical, emotional, and cognitive development. This influences all aspects of their care, from pharmacodynamics and pharmacokinetics of drugs to their communication skills and their understanding of their disease and death.

Care at home

Most children with a life limiting disease are cared for at home. Parents are both part of the team caring for the sick child and part of the family and needing care themselves. As their child's primary carers, they must be included fully in the care team—provided with information, able to negotiate treatment plans, taught appropriate skills, and assured that advice and support is accessible 24 hours a day.

Assessing symptoms

Assessing symptoms is an essential step in developing a plan of management. Often a picture must be built up through discussion with the child, if possible, combined with careful observations by parents and staff. There are formal assessment tools for assessing pain in children that are appropriate for different ages and developmental levels, but assessment is more difficult for other symptoms and for preverbal and developmentally delayed children.

Numbers of children with life limiting illness

Annual mortality from life limiting illnesses
- 1 per 10 000 children aged 1-17 years

Prevalence of life limiting illnesses
- 10 per 10 000 children aged 0-19 years

In a health district of 250 000 people, with a child population of about 50 000, in one year
- 5 children are likely to die from a life limiting illness—Cancer (2), heart disease (1), other (2)
- 50 children are likely to have a life limiting illness, about half of whom will need palliative care at any time

---

Groups of life limiting diseases in children

Group	Examples
Diseases for which curative treatment may be feasible but may fail	Cancer
Diseases in which premature death is anticipated but intensive treatment may prolong good quality life	Cystic fibrosis HIV infection and AIDS
Progressive diseases for which treatment is exclusively palliative and may extend over many years	Batten disease Mucopolysaccharidoses
Conditions with severe neurological disability that, although not progressive, lead to vulnerability and complications likely to cause premature death	Severe cerebral palsy

---

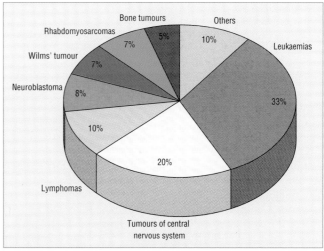

Figure 12.1   Range of malignant disease found in children

Methods of assessing pain in children
- Body charts
- Faces scales
- Numeric scales
- Diaries
- Colour tools
- Visual analogue scales
- Observation of behaviour

It is also important to consider the contribution of psychological and social factors for a child and family and to inquire about their coping strategies, relevant past experiences, and their levels of anxiety and emotional distress.

Managing symptoms

Many of the symptoms that children suffer and the approaches to relieving them have not been studied formally. Until definitive information becomes available, treatment is often based on clinical experience and adapted from general paediatric practice and palliative care of adults.

Many of the drug doses and routes used in palliative care are not licensed for children, and responsibility lies with the clinician prescribing them. In all situations the management plan should consider both pharmacological and psychological approaches along with practical help.

Children often find it difficult to take large amounts of drugs, and complex regimens may not be possible. Doses should be calculated according to a child's weight. Oral drugs should be used if possible, and children should be offered the choice between tablets, whole or crushed, and liquids. Long acting preparations are helpful, reducing the number of tablets needed and simplifying care at home. If an alternative route is needed some children find rectal drugs acceptable; they can be particularly useful in the last few days of life. Otherwise, a subcutaneous infusion can be established or, if one is in situ, a central intravenous line can be used. Parents are usually willing and able to learn to refill and load syringes and even to resite needles.

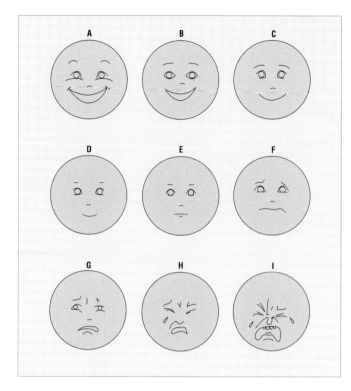

Figure 12.2   Faces scale used to measure pain effect in children (adapted from McGrath P.. *Pain in children. Nature, assessment and treatment.* New York:Guildford Press, 1990)

Specific problems

Pain

The myths perpetuating the undertreatment of pain in children have now been rejected. However, most doctors lack experience in using strong opioids in children, which often results in excess caution. The World Health Organisation's three step ladder of analgesia is equally relevant for children, with paracetamol, dihydrocodeine, and morphine sulphate forming the standard steps.

Opioids—Laxatives need to be prescribed regularly with opioids, but children rarely need antiemetics. Itching with opioids in the first few days is quite common and responds to antihistamines if necessary. Many children are sleepy initially, and parents should be warned of this lest they fear that their child's disease has suddenly progressed. Respiratory depression with strong opioids used in standard doses is not a problem in children over 1 year old, but in younger children starting doses should be reduced.

Adjuvant analgesics—Non-steroidal anti-inflammatory drugs are often helpful for musculoskeletal pains in children with non-malignant disease. Caution is needed in children with cancer and infiltration of the bone marrow because of an increased risk of bleeding. Neuropathic pain may be helped by antiepileptic and antidepressant drugs. Pain from muscle spasms can be a major problem for children with neurodegenerative diseases and may be helped by benzodiazepines and baclofen. Headaches from raised intracranial pressure associated with brain tumours are best managed with gradually increasing analgesics. Although corticosteroids are often helpful initially, the symptoms soon recur and increasing doses are needed. The considerable side effects of corticosteroids in children—rapid weight gain, changed body image, and mood swings—usually outweigh the benefits. Headaches from leukaemic deposits in the central nervous system respond well to intrathecal methotrexate.

Children and pain

- Children's nervous systems do perceive pain
- Children do experience pain
- Children do remember pain
- Children are not more easily addicted to opioids
- There is no correct amount of pain or analgesia for a given injury

Analgesic doses

Paracetamol
- Oral dose 15 mg/kg every 4-6 hours
- Rectal dose 20 mg/kg every 6 hours
- Maximum dose 90 mg/kg/24 hours, 60 mg/kg/24 hours in neonates

Dihydrocodeine
- Age <4 years 500 µg/kg orally every 4-6 hours
- Age 4-12 years 500-1000 µg/kg orally every 4-6 hours

Morphine
Immediate release preparations
- Age <1 year 150 µg/kg orally every 4 hours
- Age 1-12 years 200-400 µg/kg orally every 4 hours
- Age >12 years 10-15 mg orally every 4 hours
- Titrate according to analgesic effect and provide laxatives

12 hourly preparations
- Age <1 year 500 µg/kg orally every 12 hours
- Age 1-12 years 1 mg/kg orally every 12 hours
- Age >12 years 30 mg orally every 12 hours
- These are guidelines to starting doses, but many patients may start at higher doses after titration with immediate release morphine preparation every 4 hours

Diamorphine
- A third of total 24 hour dose of oral morphine
- Subcutaneous 24 hour infusion

Feeding

Being unable to nourish their child causes parents great distress and often makes them feel that they are failing as parents. Sucking and eating are part of children's development and provide comfort, pleasure, and stimulation. These aspects should be considered alongside a child's medical and practical problems with eating. Children with neurodegenerative disorders or brain tumours are particularly affected. In general, nutritional goals aimed at restoring health are secondary to comfort and enjoyment, although assisted feeding, via a nasogastric tube or gastrostomy, may be appropriate for those with slowly progressive disease.

Nausea and vomiting

These are common problems. Antiemetics can be selected according to their site of action and the presumed cause of the nausea. In resistant cases combining a number of drugs that act in different ways or adding a $5-HT_3$ antagonist can be helpful. Vomiting from raised intracranial pressure should be managed with cyclizine in the first instance.

Neurological problems

Watching a child have a seizure is extremely frightening for parents, and they should always be warned if it is a possibility and advised about management. A supply of rectal diazepam at home is valuable for managing seizures. Subcutaneous midazolam can enable parents to keep a child with severe repeated seizures at home. Children with neurodegenerative disease will often already be taking maintenance antiepileptic drugs, and the dose and drugs may need adjusting as the disease progresses.

Agitation and anxiety may reflect a child's need to express his or her fears and distress. Drugs such as benzodiazepines, methotrimeprazine, and haloperidol may help to provide relief, especially in the final stages of life.

Support for the family

The needs of children with a life threatening illness and their families are summarised in the report by ACT and the Royal College of Paediatrics and Child Health. Families need support from the time of diagnosis and throughout treatment as well as when the disease is far advanced. Professionals must be flexible in their efforts to help. Each family and individual within a family is unique, with different strengths and coping skills. The needs of sibling and grandparents should be included.

The family of a child with an inherited condition have additional difficulties. They may have feelings of guilt and blame, and they will need genetic counselling and information about prenatal diagnosis in the future. When an illness does not present until some years after birth several children in the same family may be affected.

Families who maintain open communication cope most effectively, but this is not everyone's pattern. Children almost always know more than their parents think, and parents should be encouraged to be as honest as they can. Play material, books, and other resources can be supplied to help with communication, and parents can be helped to recognise their children's non-verbal cues.

Sick children need the opportunity to maintain their interests and to have short term goals for as long as possible. Education is an essential part of this, as it represents their normal pattern and continues relationships with their peers. Providing information and support to teachers facilitates this.

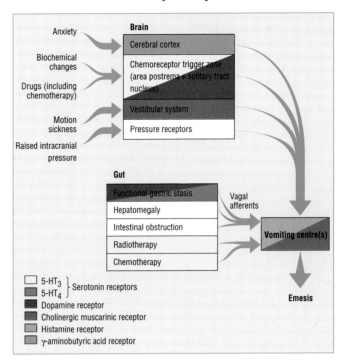

Figure 12.3 The emetic process–pathways of emesis and the neurotransmitters involved

Uses of antiemetic drugs

Cause of vomiting	Treatment
Raised intracranial pressure and sensory stimuli via cerebral cortex	Cyclizine Ondansetron Dexamethasone (only in resistant cases)
Drugs and biochemical upset	Phenothiazines Metoclopramide Domperidone Ondansetron Haloperidol
Gastrointestinal tract stimuli	Metoclopramide Domperidone Ondansetron

Support that every child and family should expect

- To receive a flexible service according to a care plan based on individual assessment of needs, with reviews at appropriate intervals
- To have a named key worker to coordinate their care and provide access to appropriate professionals
- To be included in the caseload of a paediatrician in their home area and have access to local clinicians, nurses, and therapists skilled in children's palliative care and knowledgeable about services provided by agencies outside the NHS
- To be in the care of an identified lead consultant paediatrician expert in individual child's condition
- To be supported in day to day management of child's physical and emotional symptoms and to have access to 24 hour care in the terminal stage
- To receive help in meeting the needs of parents and siblings, both during child's illness and during death and bereavement
- To be offered regular respite, including nursing care and symptom management, ranging from parts of a day to longer periods
- To be provided with drugs, oxygen, specialised feeds, and all disposable items such as feeding tubes, suction catheters, and stoma products through a single source
- To be provided with adaptations to housing and specialist equipment for use at home and school in an efficient and timely manner without recourse to several agencies
- To be helped in procuring benefits, grants, and other financial assistance

Bereavement

Grief after the death of a child is described as the most painful and enduring. It is also associated with a higher risk of pathological grief. Parents suffer multiple losses. Siblings suffer too and may have difficulty adjusting; they often feel isolated and neglected, as their parents can spare little energy or emotion for them.

Helping the bereaved family involves

- Support and assessment through the tasks of normal mourning—Most families do not need specialist counselling but benefit from general support and reassurance, supplied if possible by those who have known the family through the illness
- Information—Such as support groups and the Child Death Helpline (freephone 0800 282986); many parents value the opportunity of talking with others who have also experienced the death of a child
- Referral for specialist bereavement counselling if needed
- Gradual withdrawal of contact.

Communicating with children about death

Factors to consider
- Child's level of understanding:
  Of illness
  Of death
  Of own situation
- Child's experience
- Family's communication pattern

Methods of communication
- Verbal • Play • Drama • Art • School work • Stories

The loss of a child

- Multiple losses for parents:
  The child who has died
  Their dreams and hopes
  Their own immortality
  Their role as parents
- Stress on marriage
- Change in family structure
- Grief of siblings and grandparents

Further reading

- ACT, Royal College of Paediatrics and Child *Health guide to the development of children's palliative care services.* 1997. Available from ACT, 65 St Michael's Hill, Bristol BS2 8DZ (Tel 0117 922 1556, Fax 0117 930 4707.)
- Royal College of Paediatrics and Child Health. *Prevention and control of pain in children: a manual for health care professionals.* London, BMJ Publishing, 1997. (Tel 0171 383 6185, Fax 0171 383 6662.)

13 Communication with patients, families, and other professionals

Ann Faulkner

There is increasing awareness of the need for effective communication in health care, particularly with people who face a frightening diagnosis and an uncertain future for themselves or someone close to them.

Recent research suggests that most patients wish to know their diagnosis and the progress of treatment and disease. This may conflict with health professionals' need to protect their patients and retain an optimistic message even when the outlook is very poor.

Effective communication depends not only on the professionals but also on patients and carers. Language may be ambivalent, leading to genuine misunderstandings, and the needs of patients and carers do not always match. This may lead to health professionals feeling as though they are "pig in the middle" as they try to meet the needs of their patient and those of relatives.

When communicating with patients and relatives about incurable and life threatening disease, health professionals should remember to give attention to the environment and the physical comfort of all concerned. Standing in a corridor or a waiting room is unsatisfactory for everyone. Taking a patient or relative to a "quiet room" to discuss painful and difficult issues has the advantage of signalling the importance of the meeting and the fact that the news may be bad. Many patients, however, prefer to be in their own bed space, with the illusion of privacy given by drawn curtains. This is because the bed and surrounding space is the patient's territory, where he or she feels most in control.

Breaking bad news

Bad news cannot be broken gently, but it can be given in a sensitive manner and at the individual's pace. Many patients are well aware of the seriousness of their situation, and this may be their reason for visiting a doctor. A screening question to check a patient's perception of the situation may also show that the need is to confirm bad news rather than break it.

If bad news has to be broken, it should be at the patients' pace so that they can indicate when they wish to stop. Some individuals will not wish to hear the whole diagnosis straight away but may be more concerned with the care that is planned. If news is given too bluntly it may lead to denial.

There is always some level of shock after bad news, so some time should be given before attempting to pick up the pieces by exploring feelings and identifying concerns.

Denial

Denial may be a valid coping mechanism for those who are unable or not yet ready to adapt to the reality of a terminal illness. It can be tested by a checking question, for example: "You say you will beat this illness. Is there any time, if only for a few moments, when you are not so sure?"

This question may be answered in a way that suggests some ambivalence, such as: "Not really. Well, sometimes, if I wake early I start to wonder ... things don't add up ... but later I realise I've been silly. The early hours are a bad time." Very seldom is denial complete, though it may seem so.

Communication problems when dealing with incurable and life threatening disease
- Breaking bad news
- Denial
- Collusion
- Difficult questions
- Emotional reactions

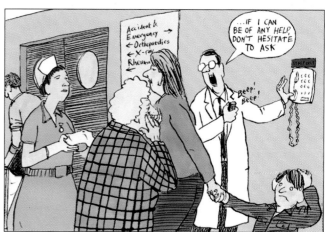

Figure 13.1

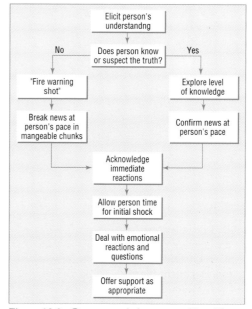

Figure 13.2 Recommended manner of breaking bad news

Denial
- May be strong coping mechanism
- Relatives may encourage
- May be total (rare)
- May be ambivalent
- Level may change over time

Patients may also indicate a total belief in the possibility of recovery, although this may change as the disease progresses. It is important to monitor changing perceptions and to explore inconsistencies.

Relatives are often happy for a patient to be in denial, for this puts off the day when painful issues have to be faced. They may argue that there is "time enough" to face reality when the patient becomes weaker.

Most patients move towards reality and will give clear indications when they are ready to talk. At this time, relatives may try to block a patient from expressing feelings by colluding to keep the truth from the patient. While acknowledging relatives' concerns, health professionals must work with the patient. It must be remembered that mentally competent adults have a right to make decisions about their own care, and it is unethical to keep the truth from patients when they are ready to face reality.

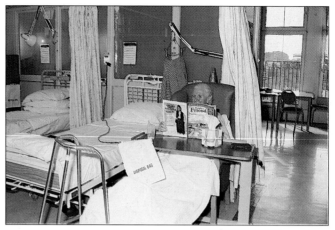

Figure 13.3   Patients may give mixed messages–reading a holiday brochure does not necessarily mean that the patient is unaware of the prognosis

Collusion

Collusion is most often seen between patients and relatives but may also occur between professionals. It is not uncommon for relatives to say, "Please don't tell him that he has got cancer." While the reasons behind this question should be explored, it is important to explain that the patient's needs for an explanation of what is happening must be met.

Collusion is generally an act of love or a need to protect another from pain. Colluders will often argue that they know the patient better than the health professionals do and know "what he can take." They may further argue that telling the truth would take away hope. Once reality has been accepted, hope can be more meaningful and based on short term, achievable goals.

Negotiation, along with acknowledging the emotional costs of collusion to carers, will generally secure access to the patient to identify his or her level of knowledge and understanding. It is very common to find that the patient is aware and also colluding, or at least suspicious of the truth, but is ready to discuss important issues.

Honest discussion allows patients to be reassured about many points of concern and helps them to be calmer and to plan and readjust hopes and aims. If collusion can be broken this can greatly enhance the quality of a patient's life and help the patient and relatives to discharge feelings and return to a more open relationship.

Difficult questions

When the reality of bad news is accepted, difficult questions—in that the answers are tenuous or constitute further bad news— may soon follow. Questions such as "How long have I got?" need exploration. A patient may have a particular aim and need to know if it is achievable. Having sought clarification, it may be possible to answer the question in relation to particular goals or aims, but specific estimations of prognosis are best avoided.

Many of these questions are rhetorical and have no clear answers. They do, however, give the questioner the opportunity to explore feelings and can help to offload major concerns. Typically, these questions are centred on a search for meaning to make sense of the current situation and may include spiritual issues and questions on religion—beliefs may be strengthened or shaken by the thought of impending death.

Dealing with collusion
- Explore reasons for collusion
- Check cost to colluder of keeping secret
- Negotiate access to patient to check their understanding of situation
- Promise not to give unwanted information
- Arrange to talk again and raise possibility of seeing couple together if both are aware of reality

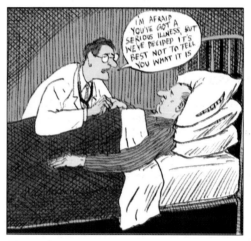

Figure 13.4

Difficult questions
- Is there a cure?
- Why me?
- How long have I got?
- What happens after this? (end of life)
- Would complementary therapies help?

Dealing with difficult questions
- Check reason for questions—for example, 'Why do you ask that now?'
- Show interest in patient's ideas—for example, 'I wonder how it looks to you?'
- Confirm or elaborate—for example, 'You are probably right,' or 'You are right in thinking that these complementary therapies don't cure, but they seem to improve some patients' quality of life'
- Be prepared to admit that you don't know—for example, 'The uncertainty must be hard to take, but I'm afraid we just don't know at this moment'
- Empathise—for example, 'Yes, it must seem unfair'

Emotional reactions

When people accept that they or someone they love will die in the near future, there are often strong emotional reactions, which need to be expressed and diffused.

In dealing with anger, health professionals should establish its cause, whether it is justified, and where it is focused. An individual can be encouraged to locate the true cause of anger rather than be allowed to displace feelings onto professionals. This can result in a healthy discharge of feelings rather than a continuation of unfocused anger. It may be that anger is felt towards a God that has "let me down." If a health professional feels unable to comment on this, a member of the clergy or a spiritual leader may help the patient feel able to express anger with his or her God.

Similarly, with guilt and blame, health professionals may not be able to take away guilt or comment when blame is apportioned, but, by exploring the particular issue with the patient, may help to put things in a more realistic perspective.

There are particular problems for professionals faced with strong emotions from patients or relatives whom they have never met before and may never meet again. This commonly occurs in accident and emergency departments and for house officers and general practitioners called to confirm a death, whether sudden or expected. It is rarely possible in this situation to fully elicit and address the issues, especially with a group of relatives. Acknowledging the emotion and thereby legitimising it, showing concern, and remaining calm will usually diffuse the immediate crisis. Such displays of emotion should not be seen as a personal attack. Others who are likely to see the relatives in the future should be informed.

Health professionals

Effective interaction with patients and carers is unlikely to be achieved in the absence of effective communication between professionals. Much is expected from doctors, nurses, and others as they deal with the problems of communicating with dying patients and their families. In communication workshops the emotional costs of caring are shown to be high, and a large proportion of these costs is related to communication within the team.

Common problems in communication between colleagues include defining roles, boundaries, and differing philosophies of care. Attempting to see problems from a colleague's point of view can enhance relationships within a team and lead to effective peer support. Regular team meetings where problems are discussed and potential solutions explored should lead to improved understanding between staff and a resultant improvement in concerted patient care.

Most areas of medicine involve palliative care, but some choose to work exclusively in this specialty. Such a choice does not necessarily assure knowledge or awareness of the emotional costs of the work. Burnout, which may not necessarily be permanent, can be the cause of conflict in interprofessional communication. In common with other specialties, adequate training, peer support, and continuing education are essential.

Major emotional reactions

Anger—Often misdirected towards health professionals
Guilt—Feelings that the illness is a punishment for past sins
Blame—Belief that current situation is fault of others

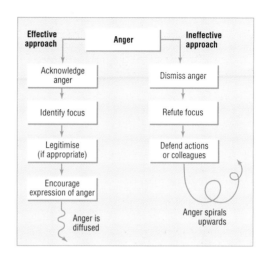

Figure 13.5   Methods of dealing with anger

Costs to professionals of dealing with dying patients and their families

- Identifying patients' concerns brings professional close to patients' pain
- Feelings of helplessness when faced with insoluble problems
- Feelings of failure when patient dies
- Imbalance between work and relaxation
- Risk of emotional burnout

Further reading

Faulkner A. *Effective interaction with patients*. 2nd ed. Edinburgh: Churchill Livingstone, 1997
Faulkner A. *When the news is bad: a guide for health professionals*. Cheltenham: Stanley Thomas. 1998.
Meredith C, Symonds P, Webster L, Pyper E, Gillis C, Fallowfield L. Information needs of patients in west Scotland: cross sectional survey of patients' views. *BMJ* 1996;313:724-6
Faulkner A, Maguire P. *Talking to cancer patients and their families*. Oxford: Oxford University Press, 1994

14   The carers

Amanda Ramirez, Julia Addington-Hall, Michael Richards

In general, most of the final year of life is spent at home, although 90% of patients spend some time in hospital and about 55% of all deaths occur there. The burdens and rewards of caring for people in their last year of life are shared between informal carers (relatives and friends or neighbours) and healthcare professionals working in institutions or in the community.

About three quarters of people receive care at home from informal carers (residential or non-residential), most of whom are women. About a third of cancer patients receive care from one close relative only, while nearly half are cared for by two or three relatives, typically a spouse and an adult child. A smaller proportion of non-cancer patients than cancer patients have access to such informal care, reflecting their older age at death.

Approximately two thirds of cancer patients and a third of non-cancer patients receive some kind of formal home nursing. District nurses are involved in the care of about half of cancer patients and a quarter of non-cancer patients. Palliative care nurse specialists, such as Macmillan nurses, are involved with about 40% of cancer patients but very few non-cancer patients. General practitioners see most patients at least five times during their last year of life, often at home. Healthcare professionals provide care on acute hospital wards and in outpatient clinics, and hospice inpatient staff care for about 17% of cancer patients during part of their terminal illness.

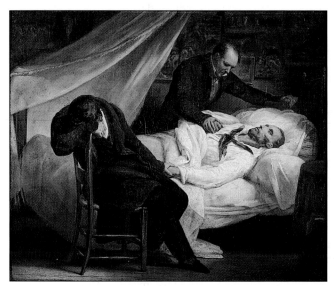

Figure 14.1   'The death of Theodore Gericault (1791-1824), with his friends Colonel Bro de Comeres and the painter' by Ary Scheffer (1795-1858). Until the start of this century, most people died at home while being cared for by family and friends

Families and friends as carers

Without the support of family and friends, it would be impossible for many patients to remain at home. It is common for families and, less often, friends to willingly take on the role of informal carer, even though this is often at considerable psychological, physical, social, and financial cost to themselves. More than half of informal carers find the caring "rewarding," 10% find it a burden, and the rest find it rewarding and burdensome in equal measure. Informal carers have a range of needs, including information and education about the patient's illness and how to care for the patient, and psychosocial support.

Information about the patient's illness
Advanced incurable illness raises difficult but important issues for health professionals to discuss with patients and their carers. Being well informed as a carer seems to allay the anxiety provoked by unnecessary uncertainty and unrealistic fears. Adequate information about the illness enables patients and carers to make informed decisions about medical care as well as broader personal and social issues.

It is no longer considered good practice to inform only relatives about a patient's disease and its management and prognosis. Exceptional circumstances may arise when patients (not relatives) clearly indicate to health professionals that they do not wish to discuss their illness or when patients are unable to understand the necessary information.

When communicating with relatives, collusion to protect patients from the truth should be discouraged. Informing only relatives can lead to mistrust and impaired communication between patients and their relatives at a time when mutual support is most needed. Patients may choose to consult with

---

Informal carers

- Most patients want to be at home during their final illness
- Informal carers are vital to the support of patients at home
- Informal carers often have unmet needs themselves
- Anxiety and depression are common among informal carers
- Many informal carers feel isolated, particularly after the patient's death

---

Needs of informal carers

Information and education about
- The patient's diagnosis
- Causes, importance, and management of symptoms
- How to care for the patient
- Likely prognosis and how the patient may die
- Sudden changes in patient's condition, particularly those which may signal that death is approaching
- What services are available and how to access them (including in emergencies)

Support during the patient's illness
- Practical and domestic
- Psychosocial
- Financial
- Spiritual

Bereavement care
(see later article on bereavement)

50

their doctor alone, but joint consultations with both patient and relatives avoid the problems that can arise when one or other party is informed first. Only between a half and two thirds of bereaved carers report having received all the information they wanted about the patient's illness.

Education about how to care for the patient

Although most informal carers have no nursing training, they perform simple nursing procedures daily. Family and friends benefit from practical instructions on how to care for patients— for example, how to lift them and how to administer drugs. There is a clear role here for district nurses and palliative care nurses. Carers describe feeling useless and helpless when they are not taught.

Psychosocial support

In the year before the death of a cancer patient, the estimated prevalence of anxiety and depression among informal carers is high—reported to be 46% for anxiety and 39% for depression. About half of carers report problems sleeping, and about a third report weight loss during the year. Carers' anxiety is rated alongside patients' symptoms as the most severe problem by both patients and families.

Professionals can encourage disclosure of carers' distress by asking questions about their perception of the patient's illness and its impact on their life. Mild psychological distress usually responds to emotional support from frontline health workers with effective communication skills. This involves explaining physical and psychological symptoms and challenging false beliefs about death and dying. In addition, carers can be encouraged to express their concerns and fears. In this way rational hope can be engendered and any sense of isolation reduced. More severe psychological distress may benefit from specialist psychological assessment and treatment.

Carers' perspective on place of death

Many patients express a desire to die at home, but carers' preferences for place of death before the event have not been established. Retrospectively, however, three quarters of bereaved carers report being satisfied with the place of death, the proportion being considerably higher when patients died at home than when they died in hospital. Excessive strain on relatives, lack of nursing staff or night sitters, and absence of equipment are common reasons why dying patients are admitted to hospital.

Healthcare professionals

Many different health professionals care for patients in their last year of life—in the community, in hospitals, and in hospices and other institutions. Some staff devote effectively the whole of their working time to palliative care, while for many others it forms only a small part of their formal workload. Unfortunately, no good information exists about this latter group, which deals with most patients with incurable disease. The following discussion is about those who work formally in palliative care.

Psychiatric morbidity and burnout

Working with patients who have incurable disease and those who are dying is widely believed to barrage staff with suffering and tragedy. However, the stress associated with caring for dying people may be counterbalanced by the satisfaction of dealing well with patients and relatives.

The prevalence of psychiatric morbidity among palliative physicians is 25%, similar to that reported by consultants

---

Failing to meet informal carers' needs

- Carers are often reluctant to disclose their needs to health professionals because they do not think it is acceptable to do so
- Reasons for this include
  Not wanting to put their needs for care before those of the patient
  Not wanting to be judged inadequate as a carer
  Believing concerns and distress are inevitable and cannot be improved
  Not being asked relevant questions by health professionals
- Attention to the needs of carers will often benefit patients—Tired and distressed carers are unlikely to give patients the physical care and emotional support they need
- A large proportion of dying patients admitted to hospital could be cared for at home if informal carers were given better support

---

Sources of support to enable informal carers to look after dying patients at home

Symptom control—General practitioners, district nurses, clinical nurse specialists such as Macmillan nurses
Nursing—Community nurses
Night sitting services—Marie Curie nurses, district nursing services
Respite care—Hospices, community hospitals
Domestic support—Social services
Information—General practitioners, district nurses, clinical nurse specialists, voluntary organisations such as BACUP
Psychosocial support—General practitioners, district nurses, Macmillan nurses, bereavement counsellors
Aids and appliances—Occupational therapists
Financial assistance—Social workers

Risk factors for psychiatric morbidity among palliative care professionals

- For senior professionals, young age or fewer years in post
- High job stress
- Low job satisfaction
- Inadequate training in communication and management skills
- Stress from other aspects of life
- Previous psychological difficulties or family history of psychiatric problems

working in specialties in acute hospitals, junior house officers, and medical students. Palliative physicians in fact report lower levels of specific work related distress or 'burnout' than other consultants.

Similarly, hospice nurses in the United States have significantly lower levels of burnout than intensive care nurses. Hospice nurses in Britain have a lower prevalence of psychiatric morbidity than Macmillan nurses and ward nurses, who in turn have a lower prevalence than district nurses and health visitors.

Job stress

The issues reported as stressful by palliative care doctors and nurses seem to be those generic to all health professionals, with overload and its effect on home life being predominant. Poor management and resource limitations, as well as issues of patient care, are also major sources of job stress.

Perhaps counterintuitively, death and dying do not emerge as a major source of job stress among either doctors working full time in palliative care or among non-specialists, including general practitioners and junior hospital doctors. Death and dying are reported as particularly stressful by palliative care nurse specialists when the patient is young, when the nurse has formed a close relationship with the patient, or when several deaths occur in a short space of time.

Nurses working in palliative care report that difficulties in their relationships with other healthcare professionals are a particular source of stress. This stress is often the result of a lack of understanding of roles and sometimes because of poorly defined roles.

Job satisfaction

Palliative physicians have significantly higher levels of job satisfaction compared with consultants working in other specialties. Helping patients through controlling symptoms and having good relationships with patients, relatives, and staff are the most highly rated sources of job satisfaction for palliative physicians.

Levels of job satisfaction are generally high among British nurses, but significantly higher among clinical nurse specialists and hospice nurses than district nurses, midwives, ward nurses, and health visitors. Clinical nurse specialists describe personal relationships with patients and their relatives and having the time to develop these as the greatest source of satisfaction in their work. Other patient related sources of satisfaction for clinical nurse specialists are controlling pain and symptoms and improving the quality of life and death for patients. Nursing dying patients and supporting their families are an important source of satisfaction as long as nurses feel that they have the time, staff, and knowledge to do it well.

Other areas of work that clinical nurse specialists describe as satisfying are relationships with colleagues and other health professionals and teamwork. This is an example of an aspect of work that can be both a major source of both stress and satisfaction.

Improving the mental health of professional carers

Maintaining and improving the mental health of professional carers is essential both for their own wellbeing and for the quality of care that they provide for patients. Strategies for improving the mental health of professionals should be implemented as a whole, so that staff are provided with both the skills and support they need to provide effective palliative care while at the same time ensuring their own emotional survival. (see the box on page 00).

Conflicts may arise in trying to meet the different needs of patients, professionals with mental health problems, and the health service as a whole. Strongly held and polarised views

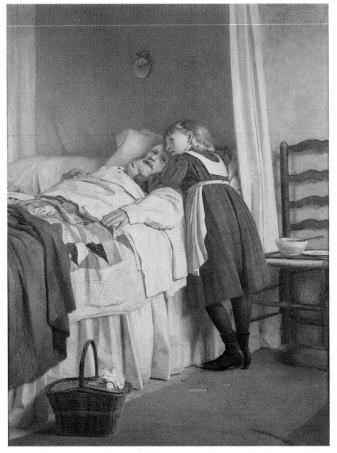

Figure 14.2 'Grandfather's little nurse' by James Hayllar (1829-1920)

Strategies for improving mental health of professionals providing palliative care

- Maintaining culture of palliative care despite the shift within health care from service to business, including
  Autonomy
  Good management
  Adequate resources, particularly with regard to workforce, so that high levels of patient care can be maintained
- Providing more effective training in
  Communication skills—Including role playing of difficult interpersonal situations with patients, relatives, and professionals
  Management skills
- Providing effective clinical supervision which addresses the physical, psychological, social, spiritual, and communication dimensions of patient care
- Providing a confidential mental health service that is independent of management and covers both personal and work related problems

---

often exist among doctors, nursing staff, and managers. Both local and more overarching initiatives are required to define and implement policies for identifying, assessing, and treating staff with mental health problems.

Identifying mental health problems

Some workers recognise that they have a mental health problem and seek advice and care from their general practitioner, a mental health colleague, or a national service (such as the BMA telephone counselling service for doctors—0645 200 169). Such professionals might be expected to have less severe mental health problems. Of more concern are those who do not refer themselves. They are identified by colleagues and should be referred to a mental health specialist in their own interests and also to the relevant service manager if there are concerns about conduct and performance that may jeopardise patient safety.

Assessment

Assessment services may either be provided within the institution where the healthcare professional works or, in order to maintain confidentiality, elsewhere by arrangement with other institutions. Such external arrangements may be particularly important for independent hospices. Assessments should be conducted by skilled mental health professionals and should include an assessment of risk to patients as well as the needs of the affected professional.

Before any assessment interview is started, an explicit discussion of confidentiality and its limits is useful. During assessment interviews, it is particularly important that professionals' health beliefs and preferences for treatment should be elicited, explored, and respected. It can be tempting to collude in self management, but this is a disservice to the professionals, who should be relieved of the burden of providing their own care.

Treatment

Treatment should ideally be provided outside the institution in which the professional works. The cornerstone of treatment is psychological therapy, either alone or in conjunction with psychotropic drugs. Choice of treatment needs to be guided by the individual case. Major factors to be considered are professionals' preferences for types of treatment and their interest in exploring and understanding their problems.

Psychological treatments delivered by trained staff are effective and include grief work, cognitive-behaviour therapy, behaviour and interpersonal therapy. Non-specific "counselling" and "support" are of limited benefit in managing complex, severe psychological problems. Many health professionals with less serious psychological problems attest to the benefit of having some form of counselling, but further evaluation is required to corroborate these anecdotal reports.

Providing mental health services to palliative care professionals

The principles are similar to those for any other group of health workers and include

- Ensuring the safety of patients
- Ensuring the optimal care of professionals
- Protecting the long term employment prospects of professionals— For the benefit of affected professionals and of the health service overall

---

Further reading

Addington-Hall JM, McCarthy M. Dying from cancer: results of a national population-based investigation. *Palliative Med* 1995; 9:295-305

Seale CF. Death from cancer and death from other causes: the relevance of the hospice approach. *Palliative Med* 1991;5:12-9

Addington-Hall JM, MacDonald LD, Anderson HR, Chamberlain J, Freeling P, Bland JM, et al. Randomized controlled trial of effects of coordinating care for terminally ill cancer patients. *BMJ* 1992; 305:1317-22

Faulkner A, Maguire P. *Talking to cancer patients and their relatives.* Oxford: Oxford Medical Publications, 1994

Graham J, Ramirez AJ, Cull A, Finlay I, Hoy A, Richards MA. Job stress and satisfaction among palliative physicians. *Palliative Med* 1996;10:185-94

---

15 Non-malignant conditions

Tony O'Brien, John Welsh, Francis G Dunn

Much medical practice is still concerned with control of symptoms rather than cure, and doctors spend considerable time palliating and modifying symptoms associated with incurable disease.

A role of specialists in palliative medicine is to offer what has been learnt about palliation of malignant disease to those caring for patients with progressive, incurable, non-malignant conditions and to share and exchange best practice. Many symptoms experienced by cancer and non-cancer patients are similar: cancer patients' symptoms may be more severe, but those of non-cancer patients tend to be more prolonged.

The approach to controlling pain in progressive non-malignant conditions can be adopted from the strategy for managing cancer related pain. After an accurate diagnosis of the pain, appropriate treatment can be started: the principles of the World Health Organisation's analgesic ladder (discussed in the first article of this series) apply equally to non-cancer patients. The strength of analgesia chosen depends on the severity of the pain, and the choice of adjuvant analgesic depends on the pathogenesis of the pain.

Doctors may be concerned about giving opioids to patients with chronic non-malignant pain. This is a justifiable worry if a systematic approach to selecting patients is not adopted. In the absence of malignancy, underprescribing of opioids for pain is not uncommon. When opioids are prescribed and effective patients, will reasonably, request regular or increased doses. Pseudoaddiction, the seeking of drugs to control pain rather than to feed psychological dependence, should be identified.

Advanced respiratory disease

The commonest chronic respiratory disorder requiring palliation is chronic obstructive pulmonary disease. Like many non-malignant conditions, however, the clinical course is not easy to predict, and a patient's life span with this condition can be decades. The illness may be characterised by frequent exacerbations followed by recovery to baseline status.

Management

If standard treatments—including oxygen, bronchodilators, antibiotics, and corticosteroids—do not adequately relieve symptoms, opioids and benzodiazepines should be considered for breathlessness.

An immediate release formulation of morphine will generally ease resistant breathlessness, but use must be judged on an individual basis. Morphine should be started at a low dose, 2.5-5.0 mg every 4 hours, and titrated to an effective dose. For patients with carbon dioxide retention, careful monitoring is vital, and the frequency of dosing may have to be reduced. If an opioid is given a laxative must also be prescribed.

Often patients are anxious, and judicious use of a low dose benzodiazepine can be helpful. Care should be exercised with diazepam as, even at low doses, it will tend to accumulate because of its long half life. Lorazepam is shorter acting.

Discussion, explanations, and planning and non-drug measures are an integral part of management. Rehabilitation is desirable when possible and should be tailored to the individual patient.

A strong body of opinion argues that the skills and philosophies of palliative care should be extended to all care settings. This is optimally delivered by those working in their own specialty—such as neurology, cardiology, and respiratory medicine. Training in basic palliative care should form part of the undergraduate and postgraduate curricula for healthcare professionals. The success and relevance of palliative care will be judged not by the number of specialist teams but by the capacity to influence the care offered to all patients irrespective of diagnosis and place of care

---

Symptoms common to malignant and non-malignant conditions

Physical
- Pain
- Breathlessness
- Anorexia
- Immobility
- Constipation

Social
- Loss of employment
- Role change
- Fear for dependants

Psychological
- Depression
- Fear and anxiety
- Uncertainty
- Guilt

Existential
- Religious
- Non-religious
- Meaning of life
- Why?

Guidelines for prescribing opioids for pain control in non-malignant conditions

- Careful assessment of patient—Liaise with others as necessary; psychologist, psychiatrist, other physicians
- Careful assessment of pain
- Encourage patient to keep a pain diary
- Apply WHO guidelines for choice of analgesia
- Care needed if previous problems with drug dependency
- Opioids should not reinforce pain behaviour
- One prescriber of opioids
- Make a contract (fixed time, conditions)
- Regular review—Of patient, pain, function, analgesia
- Assess opioid responsiveness of pain
- Overall quality of life should improve
- Function should improve—Can range from improved concentration or enjoyment to substantial increase in mobility

Advanced cardiac disease

The management of cardiac disease at all stages has a substantial palliative component, and, unlike management of cancer, there are few opportunities for cure. This section focuses on palliative care in cardiac failure, as this is the final common pathway in most patients with advanced cardiac disease who do not die suddenly.

Prevalence—Cardiac failure affects 1-2% of the adult population, and the prevalence rises steeply with age (to more than 10% of those aged over 70). It is a disabling and lethal condition that also has a detrimental effect on quality of life. Up to 30% of affected patients require hospitalisation in any year (120 000 admissions annually in the United Kingdom). Mortality is higher than in many forms of cancer, with a 60% annual mortality with grade 4 heart failure and an overall five year mortality of 80% in men.

Clinical aspects—There are several important similarities to and differences from cancer. The now seldom used term cardiac cachexia is as apposite a term in 1997 as it was 40 years ago. Advances in antianginal therapy and interventional techniques have reduced the importance of pain as a dominant feature of cardiac failure.

Management
General
Patients with advanced cardiac failure will be faced with frequent admissions to hospital. Since patients much prefer home management if possible, this should be recognised. Cardiac liaison nurses similar to the highly developed Macmillan system would reduce the number of admissions by early detection of worsening clinical features and by ensuring that patients' homes met all the necessary requirements.

Current indications for hospital admission are
- Need for intravenous therapy
- Persistent paroxysmal nocturnal breathlessness and orthopnoea
- Refractory dependent oedema, despite up to 120 mg oral frusemide twice daily
- Symptomatic postural hypotension
- Fluid leakage from lower limbs
- Development of dysrhythmias.

Dietary advice is important since patients may be obese or cachectic. Frequent small meals are preferred, which should be tailored to each patient's tastes. Tumour necrosis factor and interleukins are implicated in the causation of cachexia, and fish oils may reduce their levels. Supplements of fat soluble and water soluble vitamins may also be necessary to counteract their increased urinary loss and reduced absorption. A small amount of alcohol may help as an appetite stimulant and anxiolytic.

Reducing fluid intake to 1500 ml a day and avoiding excessively salty foods (but not to the extent of making food tasteless) will help in controlling oedema. There is evidence that exercise may lessen breathlessness and improve both quality of life and psychological wellbeing. This must be tailored to patients' individual needs.

Drug treatment
The main emphasis is symptom relief: drugs being given to improve prognosis should be reviewed.

Opioids, combined with antiemetic drugs if necessary, are useful for control of nocturnal breathlessness.

Diuretics also have a key role—orally, intravenously, or in combination depending on the severity of fluid retention. However, awareness of the clinical and biochemical features of overdiuresis is necessary. This can lead to postural

---

Clinical aspects of cardiac failure compared with cancer

Similarities to cancer	Differences from cancer
● Breathlessness, lethargy, cachexia	● Pain not a major problem
● Nausea, anorexia, abnormal taste	● Oedema a more dominant feature with a different mechanism
● Weight loss (loss of muscle mass countered by fluid retention)	
● Constipation	● Predicting life expectancy less easy
● Poor mobility	● Less need for opioids
● Insomnia, confusion, depression	● Patients mistakenly perceive it as a more benign condition than malignancy
● Dizziness, postural hypotension, cough	
● Jaundice, susceptibility to infection	● Anaemia not usually present
● Polypharmacy	
● Abnormal liver function tests	
● Fear of the future	

Home care for advanced cardiac failure
- Assess appropriateness of the home—Such as comfortable bed or recliner chair, easy access to toilet, family support
- Establish need for oxygen therapy—Balance benefits and risks
- Monitor fluid status and appropriateness of diuretic treatment
- Consider quick release oral morphine 5 mg at night to ease breathlessness
- For night sedation consider temazepam 10-20 mg or, in elderly people, thioridazine 10 mg or haloperidol 0.5 mg
- Assess need for dietary advice, particularly to ensure adequate energy intake
- Ensure optimum treatment of heart failure provided drugs are not causing symptoms
- Regularly consider need for hospital admission

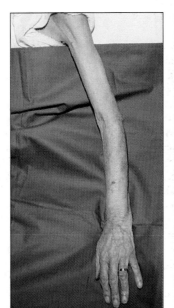
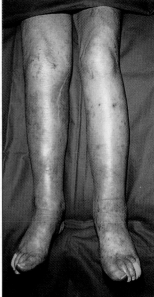

Figure 15.1   Marked muscle wasting in the arms (left) combined with oedema of the legs (right) in a patient with advanced heart failure

hypotension, though other causes exist, some of which are shared by patients with cancer.

Digoxin has known symptomatic benefit in advanced heart failure. The optimal dose which avoids toxicity must be found.

Angiotensin converting enzyme inhibitors are of symptomatic benefit, and the dose should be titrated to ensure maximum benefit without adverse effects. Since many patients are volume depleted and hypotensive, small supervised test doses should be given—such as 6.25 mg captopril after 12-24 hours without diuretics. In patients unable to take angiotensin converting enzyme inhibitors other vasodilators should be considered.

Sublingual glyceryl trinitrate is helpful during episodes of breathlessness.

Vaccination—Influenza and pneumococcal vaccination are worth considering despite the advanced nature of the disease.

Counselling and psychological support

The highly developed support network for cancer patients is not available to patients with end stage cardiac disease. Counselling is certainly challenging in this situation because of the high incidence of sudden death (up to 50%) and the misconception of patients, who underestimate the seriousness of the situation. Application of many of the principles of palliative care is needed to optimise this aspect of management.

Causes of postural hypotension in terminal cardiac disease and cancer

Cardiac related
- Diuretics
- Vasodilators

Cancer related
- Opioids
- Antidepressants
- Adrenal insufficiency due to metastasis

Common to both
- Bed rest
- Coexistent disease
- Muscle wasting and poor venous tone
- Reduced fluid intake and vomiting

The future of palliation in advanced cardiac disease
- Development of clinical specialist home support nurses to reduce need for hospital admission
- Improved understanding of mechanisms and treatment of nausea and cachexia
- Better early detection and control of oedema
- Improved recognition of need for psychological support and counselling

---

Symptomatic management of advanced heart failure

Breathlessness
- Oxygen
- Opioids—Regular, quick release oral morphine 5 mg, or intravenous diamorphine 2.5 mg if acutely distressed
- Non-drug measures—Such as fan, positioning, explanation, reassurance
- Diuretics, digoxin
- Vasodilators

Muscle wasting
- Physiotherapy
- Assess diet and energy intake

Fatigue
- Reassess drug therapy

Lightheadedness
- Check for postural hypotension
- Check for drug induced hypotension, from vasodilator or diuretic

Nausea, abnormal taste, anorexia
- Check drug treatments
- Check liver function
- Frequent small meals
- Appetite stimulants such as alcohol
- Consider metoclopramide

Oedema
- Early detection important
- Loop diuretics—Frusemide remains first choice
- Restrict fluid intake to 1.5-2 litres a day
- Mild salt restriction—No salt added at table
- Bed rest in early stages—If out of bed raise lower limbs via foot stool or recliner chair
- Aim for weight loss of 0.5-1 kg a day
- Combination diuretic treatments may be needed—Such as metolazone 2.5 mg on alternate days or bendrofluazide 5 mg/day plus frusemide
- Monitor electrolytes

Advanced neurological disease

Specialist palliative care services have developed a particular expertise in managing patients with progressive and advanced neurological conditions, of which motor neurone disease is perhaps the best studied example. Motor neurone disease (amyotrophic lateral sclerosis) is a disabling disorder of unknown aetiology for which there is no known cure. The mean survival is typically about three to four years.

Motor neurone disease can evoke the most negative attitudes in many medical staff, which are quite often conveyed to patients and their families. However, many of its symptoms can be alleviated by strict attention to detail and applying well established principles. While motor neurone disease is comparatively rare, many of its symptoms are common to other chronic neurological conditions. Patients with motor neurone disease require input from a range of disciplines. A strong commitment to teamwork is needed, and efficient channels of communication must be established and maintained.

The prevalence of symptoms in patients with motor neurone disease is similar to that in cancer patients. In a sample of patients referred to a hospice many of the cancer patients were referred specifically for symptom control, compared with only 15% of patients with motor neurone disease, all of whom had multiple symptoms.

Specialists involved in caring for patients with motor neurone disease
- Neurologist
- Neurophysiologist
- Palliative medicine physician
- Endoscopist
- Anaesthetist
- Surgeon
- Respiratory physician
- General practitioner
- Physiotherapist
- Occupational therapist
- Speech and language therapist
- Nutritionist or dietician
- Nursing staff
- Social worker
- Patient support groups

Adapted from Smith AM, Eve A, Sykes NP. Palliative care services in Britain and Ireland 1990—an overview. *Palliat Med* 1992;6:277-91

Symptoms of patients on admission to a hospice

	Patients with motor neurone disease (n=124)	Patients with cancer (n=809)
Constipation	81 (65%)	338 (48%)
Pain	71 (57%)	558 (69%)
Cough	66 (53%)	380 (47%)
Insomnia	59 (48%)	235 (29%)
Breathlessness	58 (47%)	405 (50%)

Adapted from: O'Brien T, Kelly M, Saunders CM. Motor neurone disease: a hospice perspective. *BMJ* 1992;304: 471-3

Management of symptoms

Pain

Pain is common and troublesome in motor neurone disease, with 65-70% of patients reporting it to be a major symptom. Pain may occur at single or multiple sites and is often described as aching, cramping, burning, and shock-like. Some of the pain is caused by the stiffness associated with prolonged immobility and will be helped by physiotherapy and passive exercises. Additional relief can be achieved with a non-steroidal anti-inflammatory drug.

Many of these pains will require a strong opioid, and oral morphine is the drug of choice. The doses required are generally quite low, and patients may be maintained on stable doses of morphine for long periods. Although the value of opioids in motor neurone disease is generally accepted, their use is sometimes inappropriately reserved for the 'terminal' phase only.

Swallowing and nutritional difficulties

Dysphagia is a common and distressing problem, and patients are often acutely embarrassed by the dribbling and coughing associated with trying to eat, while their carers are often frustrated by how long it takes to complete a meal. Salivary dribbling will usually respond to an anticholinergic agent. If drugs are unsuccessful, radiotherapy should be considered in order to dry up salivary secretions.

The swallowing reflex is often so impaired that patients cannot maintain an adequate fluid and energy intake. They will probably have experimented with a range of foods of varying consistencies, often supplemented by high energy drinks. Despite this they feel hungry and thirsty, and at least part of their continued clinical deterioration is related to their poor nutritional status.

Nasogastric tube feeding is unpleasant and cumbersome and is generally not well tolerated. Early consideration should be given to nutritional support with percutaneous endoscopic gastrostomy tube feeding. Improved nutritional status will result in a greater sense of wellbeing and should enhance patients' quality of life. Each patient will require careful explanation of the procedure and will need ongoing information and support. Complications are rare, with a mortality of 0.3-1.0% and morbidity of 3.0-5.9%.

Respiratory complications

These are a major source of morbidity and mortality in patients with motor neurone disease. Most deaths are associated with catastrophic respiratory muscle weakness. Symptoms such as cough and breathlessness are very common and may be evident at first diagnosis. Routine assessment of pulmonary function, when interpreted in conjunction with symptoms, can provide a useful indicator of disease progression and prognosis.

Management involves a multidisciplinary approach with careful assessment, explanation, and reassurance. Correct positioning enables patients to derive maximum benefit from weakened muscle groups. Oral morphine or low dose diazepam often helps to reduce the subjective sensation of breathlessness. Respiratory tract infections are sometimes difficult to diagnose clinically because of impaired inspiratory effort: symptomatic infections should be treated with appropriate antibiotics.

Ventilatory support is often controversial, yet many patients and families cope admirably with home ventilation and derive great symptomatic benefit and maintain an acceptable quality of life. Ventilatory support should be undertaken only after a comprehensive multidisciplinary assessment. Patients must be fully aware of all that is involved and be assured of adequate support.

Management of symptoms of motor neurone disease

Cough—Methadone linctus 2 mg/5 ml twice daily
Constipation—Combined purgative and softening laxative
Insomnia—Temazepam 10-20 mg, haloperidol 0.5 mg, thioridazine 10-75 mg
Difficulty swallowing oral secretions—Hyoscine butylbromide or hyoscine hydrobromide patch
Poor mobility—Physiotherapy

Response of patients with motor neurone disease to opioids

	Good	Fair	No response
Breathlessness (n = 59)	48 (81%)	2 (3%)	3 (5%)
Pain (n = 49)	36 (74%)	9 (18%)	0

Adapted from: O'Brien T, Kelly M, Saunders CM. Motor neurone disease: a hospice perspective. *BMJ* 1992;304: 471-3

> **Percutaneous endoscopic gastrostomy feeding is indicated for those patients who feel hungry or thirsty or who are unable to consume sufficient calories to meet their metabolic needs**

Complications of percutaneous endoscopic gastrostomy

- Wound infection
- Peritonitis
- Septicaemia
- Peristomal leakage
- Tube dislodgement
- Aspiration
- Bowel perforation
- Gastrocolic fistula

16 Care in the community

Bill O'Neill, Ann Rodway

The physical complexities of progressive and life threatening disease, coupled with attendant emotional and psychological consequences, demand careful coordination between primary, secondary, and tertiary care. Across the whole range of health services, an increasing amount of care is being provided on an outpatient basis or independently of hospitals altogether: most terminally ill patients spend most of their time at home.

In the planning of care and agreeing a management plan, patients must be given an opportunity to express their wishes and these must be taken into account. Patients can make valid choices between treatment options only if they know what is happening, what help is available, what is likely to happen, and what help will be available in the future.

It is important to document accurately at each point what a patient's wishes are. Information must be tailored to patients to meet their need for knowledge and given at a pace with which they can cope. Rarely, patients may choose not to be informed. Some patients may wish to complete an advance statement, giving instructions about their wishes in the event of their losing the capacity to decide or to communicate.

Demands of home care

It can be much easier to care for patients in a hospital, hospice, or nursing home because of the infrastructure and immediate support available. Caring for a patient at home presents a challenge, and sometimes a burden, that is not as easily shared as in an institutional setting.

Although most patients wish to die at home, barely a quarter manage to do so. Over 90% of all patients with cancer spend some time in hospital during the last year of life, while 55% die in hospital and 17% die in a hospice. The desired place of death may change with altered circumstances, the most obvious being difficult symptoms and lack of practical help at home. Patients who are frightened, insecure, or lack confidence in their support network are more likely to seek urgent admission to hospital or hospice. Equally, if informal carers are physically or mentally tired they are more likely to seek admission, even when death is imminent.

Managing a patient at home requires not only an accurate assessment of the patient and his or her illness, concomitant physical and psychological symptoms, and support network but also an assessment of the patient's home. This may require an occupational therapist or physiotherapist to advise on the need for aids and, if necessary, modifications to the home. Forward planning is crucial, and much effort has to go into the general structure of care, which must be individualised for each patient. While primary care teams can systematically work through the aspects noted above, there is no automatic formula for all cases.

Stressed families caring for a dying patient are unlikely to have their thoughts well organised at the time of a first meeting. Primary care teams should help families and patients to evolve their thoughts, feelings, anxieties, and fears so that they can verbalise them, discuss what needs to be discussed, find answers to those problems that have solutions, get reassurance when it is appropriate, and develop a plan of action for problems that have no easy solution and are likely to worsen.

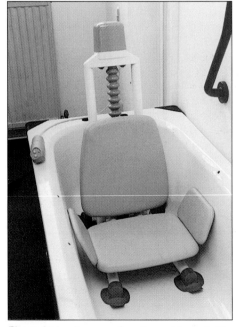

Figure 16.1   A range of equipment is available for fitting to a standard domestic bath

Life threatening disease often exposes ambiguities in family relationships. General practitioners are in an excellent position to understand past and present relationships, but they can be surprised by old unresolved problems uncovered in the stress of a terminal illness. An understanding of past relationships and behaviours, coupled with discussion and explanation of what is happening, may ease the situation. More complex problems may require referral to a clinical psychologist or a professional trained in family therapy. However, do not expect to resolve 30 years of conflict in the three weeks before death.

Primary care teams must maintain a role as gatekeepers to care, not just for referrals to specialist centres but also for referrals to specialist teams in the community. General practitioners should be consulted before hospital patients are referred to specialist community teams prior to discharge. Timing of referral is important, and, while referrals should be made early rather than late, there should be explicit agreement on the extent of involvement, including responsibility for counselling and emotional support for patient and family.

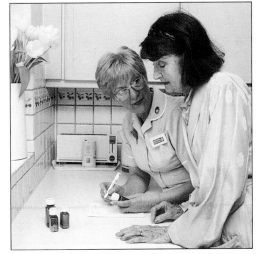

Figure 16.2 Many specialist nurses provide detailed advice and recommendations on drug therapy, a task that was previously the exclusive remit of doctors

Coordination of professionals

Communication

If a patient is to be cared for at home, good communication from hospital or hospice to primary care team is essential. Practical difficulties make it harder to achieve high standards of communication in the community and between institutional and community staff than within institutions.

Some primary care teams allow specialist community teams access to records held at the practice. Others invite members of community teams to practice meetings when patient care is being discussed. There is an argument for patient held records, in which details of proposed treatment and any subsequent changes could be recorded. Community nursing notes are commonly kept in patients' homes, and it is important that others caring for patients should consult these notes and make entries in them in order to facilitate communication.

Advances in information technology and the resolution of concerns about confidentiality and security of data offer opportunities for sharing computerised records so that all those treating a patient have immediate access to details of treatment and any investigations performed.

Teamwork

Effective teamwork requires mutual understanding of the roles and responsibilities of each member of the team. General practitioners must maintain overall responsibility for the medical care of patients at home. Depending on patients' particular needs, the delivery of care is shared with the various members of the primary care team and members of the community team. District nurses play a key role when nursing care is required.

Regrettably, many patients have to be admitted to hospital or hospice because of inadequate practical help at home. Many families are disillusioned by the 'package of care' provided. Needs are often not met—a common example is that even frequent visits by district nurses cannot always coincide with the needs of a patient to use the commode or toilet or to be turned in bed. Informal carers, particularly those looking after a patient single handed, find this very difficult and frustrating, especially when it results in admission to hospital or hospice. The ability to mobilise support often depends on local resources but also on organisation and structure.

> **Accurate and clear information must be rapidly available to primary care teams about the disease, treatment, expected events, likely prognosis, what the patient has asked and has been told, and who should be contacted if a problem arises**

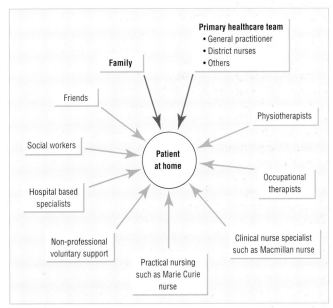

Figure 16.3 Groups involved in delivery of care to terminally ill patients at home

> **Complex rotas of visiting arrangements may be required, particularly for patients who are living alone, and these may involve social workers, home helps, district nurses, specialist palliative care nurses, and night sitters. The rota of care may include support from neighbours and other voluntary help**

Nursing services

The availability of nursing services varies widely. In some areas district nursing services are limited to daytime, but available seven days a week; in others there is a twilight service; while in others a 24 hour on call service is provided. High dependency care may require a night sitting service, which can be provided by care assistants or by trained registered nurses. The choice may depend on the complexity of care and the need for drugs to be administered. Some health authorities have contracts for a service provided by Marie Curie nurses specially trained in the care of dying patients.

Palliative care teams

Most districts in Britain now have palliative care teams based in the community to advise and support primary care teams and patients and their families. The composition of these teams varies. All have specialist palliative care nurses (also known as Macmillan nurses), with varying levels of medical and other support. Some are attached to hospices and other specialist inpatient units. Many specialist nurses provide detailed advice and recommendations on drug therapy, a task that was previously the exclusive remit of doctors.

Financial and legal help

The greatest difficulties often arise in the boundaries between health and social care. The responsibilities of social workers in the community will include assessment for a 'package of care' and, when appropriate, assessment for residential or nursing home care.

Although this is not always accepted by social services staff, many healthcare workers assume that financial and legal advice should be provided via a social worker. Patients and families may benefit from advice on access to benefits such as disability living allowance (DLA) and mobility allowance. Some patients and families find it necessary to supplement the care provided by statutory services with paid help, and this may warrant a claim for disability living allowance. Many patients need help in completing the forms required.

Macmillan Cancer Relief and other charities provide grants to patients with terminal diseases for specific purposes—help with paying electricity or gas bills, paying for the installation of a telephone so that patients have access to emergency support, home equipment such as a food liquidiser for those with difficulty swallowing, and the provision of bed linen.

Attendance at specialist clinics

For some patients, such as those presenting with advanced lung cancer, the diagnosis may be made after a single outpatient visit and procedure. Depending on the symptoms, no further hospital attendance may be indicated. Effective medical care at home depends on the role of the patient's general practitioner and the avoidance of unnecessary outpatient visits, which serve to perpetuate the sharp divide between hospital and community care.

At all stages of disease, there is a need to demystify the care provided in hospital, and for each visit the reviewing doctor should carefully consider whether it is justified. In some situations continuing hospital attendance may be appropriate as long as the patient is able and wishes this—for example, a patient who benefits from recurrent abdominal paracentesis for ascites or who needs three weekly infusions of bisphosphonates to prevent recurrence of hypercalcaemia of malignancy.

An efficient model of care should include arrangements for general practitioners to plan specialist outpatient visits at short notice. Visits made solely for a blood test or to allow hospital staff to check on the progression of disease should be avoided.

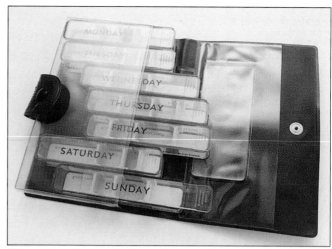

Figure 16.4 Some patients require complex drug regimens, in which case pills can be laid out in a dosette box by a family member or community nurse

---

Disability living allowance for patients with a prognosis of less than six months

- There is a fast track system for access to disability living allowance which obviates the need for assessment by a doctor appointed by the Department of Social Security
- In addition to the standard form, a further form (DS1500) must be completed and signed by a doctor

---

Macmillan Cancer Relief and patient welfare

In addition to providing medical nursing and social support for patients with cancer, Macmillan Cancer Relief has five caseworkers in its patient welfare department offering help and advice to healthcare workers on grant applications by patients

Caseworkers for different regions in the United Kingdom can be contacted on the telephone numbers below

- Scotland, Wales, and Northern Ireland   0171 867 9492
- North of England   0171 867 9493
- Midlands   0171 867 9490
- South and south west   0171 867 9491
- London and south east   0171 867 9496

Questions to ask about patients' visits to hospital

- What were the benefits of the visit?
- What were the negative features of the visit?
- Was this a justified visit?
- Who else is seeing this patient?
- What does the patient want?
- Has the situation been communicated properly with the general practitioner?

Emergencies

Emergencies (the subject of an earlier article in this series) are among the most challenging aspects of palliative care in the community. Primary health care teams should give clear, unambiguous advice about who should be contacted in an emergency. The advice should be agreed by all agencies caring for a patient, and there should be clear understanding of who should be called and how they can be contacted and a general discussion of the situations that may herald an emergency.

It may be appropriate to leave supplies of drugs in a patient's home for emergency use by community nursing staff and possibly family carers. Many patients are terrified of having uncontrolled symptoms overnight or at weekends, and a supply of suitable drugs may help to allay this fear.

Arrangements should made for general practitioners, district nurses, and other community health workers to have access at all times to specialist advice from consultants in palliative medicine, pain, oncology, and surgery. Advice alone is often sufficient, but in some cases emergency outpatient assessment or home visits will be needed.

Foreseeable emergencies

Some emergencies can be anticipated, and appropriate arrangements made. Decisions should be taken on whether patients and their family carers should be advised of the risk of sudden bleeding, convulsions, or other potentially catastrophic events. The amount of information given will depend on the illness and its likely progress, the probability of an emergency occurring, the patient's wish for information, the family's need for information, and the support available immediately on site.

District nurses and specialist nurses, as well as general practitioners, should be aware of the importance of changes in symptoms that herald emergencies. Patients should be advised to report the development of muscular weakness or difficulties with bowel or bladder control, which could indicate spinal cord compression.

Respite care

Respite care can take the form of increased support in the home or attendance at a day centre, perhaps even once a week. The latter has the additional benefit of providing a change of environment, which is stimulating for the patient.

The range of services available at day centres varies greatly. Some are modelled on outpatient hospital departments, and arrangements can be made for treatments such as intravenous infusion of bisphosphonates or blood transfusion. Others, based on nursing care, can provide changes of dressings, treatment of lymphoedema, and more basic nursing needs such as access to an assisted bath. Others are based on recreational and diversional therapy, occasionally with additional services such as those of a hairdresser.

Inpatient respite care may be provided in inpatient units managed by general practitioners, hospices, or hospitals. During these admissions there is time to reassess symptoms, both physical and non-physical, and to attempt rehabilitation if appropriate. A common assumption is that patients with advancing cancer naturally "take to their bed," despite the fact that many patients benefit enormously from physiotherapy, occupational therapy, and other rehabilitative support.

Respite facilities are offered by certain nursing homes that admit patients on a temporary basis. Macmillan Cancer Relief and other charities may finance a week of respite care in nursing homes and residential holiday homes.

Drugs for emergencies in palliative care

- Diamorphine (or morphine) ampoules 10 mg or 30 mg
- Midazolam ampoules 10 mg
- Methotrimeprazine ampoules 50 mg
- Haloperidol ampoules 5 mg
- Hyoscine hydrobromide ampoules 0.6 mg

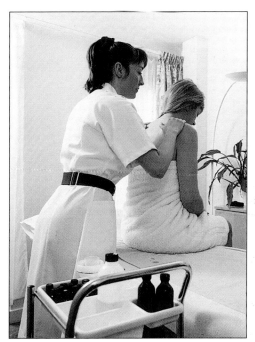

Figure 16.5 In addition to conventional treatment, some outpatient and day centres offer a range of complementary therapies

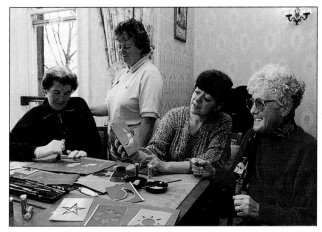

Figure 16.6 Occupational therapy at a Marie Curie centre

Death in the community

If death is anticipated and likely to occur at home it is important that the patient and family carers have an opportunity to discuss any anxieties that they may have about this. Many carers will never have been present at a death or seen a dead body, having been shielded from the death of parents, grandparents, or other relatives. Any impressions or experience they have may be based on violent or distressing deaths in films or on television.

While emergencies resulting in sudden death are not uncommon, the mode of death of many terminally ill patients can be anticipated. An explanation of progressive loss of consciousness and awareness, and of how any pain or breathlessness can be treated, will lessen many anxieties. Care must be taken not to make promises that cannot be fulfilled—promising total relief of pain or breathlessness that cannot then be achieved is likely to lessen confidence and cause difficulties in the future care of the patient and of surviving relatives.

After death

When given the opportunity many relatives ask about what will happen after death—what care is required for the body, who should be informed, and what procedures must be undertaken. In advising patients of the requirements after death, it is usually sufficient to explain the need for certification and registration of the death and to assure them that when they contact a funeral undertaker they will get all the necessary support and advice. Many undertakers provide written information for bereaved relatives, and information is also available from the Department of Social Security.

The responsibility for notifying a death to the registrar rests with a relative or, in the absence of a relative, a person present at the death or the owner of the premises in which the death has taken place. A doctor who attended the patient during his or her last illness will normally issue a medical certificate of the cause of death or report the death to the coroner. If the body is to be buried there is no legal requirement for it to be seen by a doctor after death, although it is advisable for the doctor who issues the certificate to do so. Some funeral directors refuse to move a body until it has been seen by a doctor and the death confirmed. In many institutions—including nursing homes, hospices, and hospitals—appropriately trained nurses can verify a death and agree to the removal of a body. The Royal College of Nursing has issued guidance on this.

If the body is to be cremated it must first be seen by the certifying doctor and by a second, independent medical practitioner whose registration is of at least five years' standing and who is not a partner or a relative of the first doctor or of the deceased. Membership of the same hospital clinical firm is interpreted as similar to partnership in general practice.

Although there is no legal obligation for care after the death of a patient, many doctors recognise their role in the care of bereaved relatives. Most palliative care teams offer a bereavement visit some time after the death, while many general practitioners also have relatives of the deceased as patients. Bereavement is the subject of the next and final article in this series.

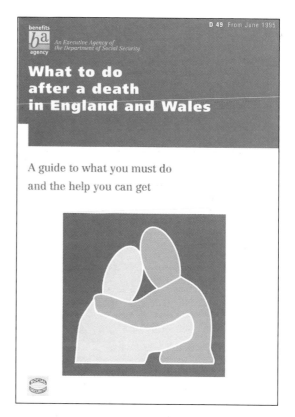

Figure 16.7 The department of Social Security provides information on the requirements after a death and on available services and benefits

---

Circumstances in which a death must be reported to the coroner

- Deceased was not attended in last illness by a doctor
- Deceased was not seen by a doctor either after death or within 14 days before death
- Cause of death is unknown
- There is any doubt about natural cause—suggestions of violence, neglect, or other suspicious circumstances
- Death was due to industrial disease or poisoning (including alcoholism)
- Death occurred during surgery or before recovery from anaesthesia (often interpreted as within 24 hours)
- Death was due to an abortion
- Death occurred in prison or in police custody

Some coroners advise that deaths that occur within 24 hours of admission to hospital and those where there is any allegation of negligence should also be reported.

Adapted from: Knight B. *Legal aspects of medical practice*. Edinburgh: Churchill Livingstone, 1992

The photograph of the bath aid and the dosette box are reproduced with permission of the Disability Living Foundation. The photographs of the specialist nurse advising on drug therapy, of the nurse providing complementary therapy, and of occupational therapy at a day centre are reproduced with permission of Marie Curie Cancer Care

17 Bereavement

Frances Sheldon

Bereavement is a universal human experience and potentially dangerous to health. It is associated with a high mortality for some groups, and up to a third of bereaved people develop a depressive illness. Help targeted at those most at risk has been shown to be effective and to make the most efficient use of scarce resources. When a death is anticipated, preparation for bereavement can be made, and this can also improve outcome.

The process of grief

Grief has been described in terms of stages or tasks, but all writers emphasise that it is not a neat and ordered process but rather overlapping phases of a mixture of emotions and responses.

A sense of shock, disbelief, and denial may occur even when death is expected, but these are likely to last longer and be more intense with an unexpected death.

During the acute distress that usually follows, bereaved people often experience physical symptoms, which may be due to anxiety or may mimic the symptoms of the deceased. For some, there may be questioning of previously deeply held beliefs, while others find great support from their faith, the rituals associated with it, and the social contact with others of a like mind, which religious affiliation often brings.

In time the great majority of bereaved people gradually re-engage with life and adjust to their situation. However, family events and anniversaries may sometimes reawaken painful memories and feelings—in this sense grief never really ends.

A crucial factor is the meaning of the loss for the bereaved person, and the painful search for understanding of why the death occurred is another common feature of bereavement. Throughout the period of bereavement bereaved people may oscillate between concentrating on the pain of the loss and distracting themselves through work or planning for the future.

Recent research suggests that men and women in western societies tend to grieve differently. Women are more emotional and loss focused: men are more inclined to work on the practical tasks that bereavement brings. If the emphasis is exclusively on one or the other, adjustment to the loss may be more difficult.

Factors associated with poor outcome

Research has identified several factors that increase the risk of poor outcome. The relationship with the deceased person is very important: an ambivalent or dependent relationship is linked with higher distress, no matter whether it was the person who died or the person bereaved who was overtly dependent on the other.

Elderly widowers in Western societies have a particularly high risk of dying in the first six months after their partner's death, and suicide risk is markedly increased in this group. Widows tend to report more symptoms in bereavement than widowers—younger widows acknowledge more psychological difficulties, older widows report more physical symptoms.

The death of a child is regarded by Western societies as one of the most painful bereavements because it is now so rare. There is a high risk of marital difficulty and breakdown for parents after a child's death.

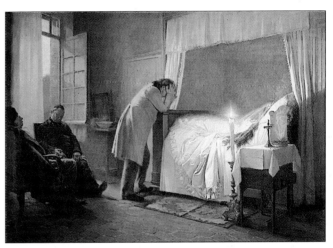

"The deathbed of Madame Bovary" by Albert-Auguste Fourie (b 1854)

Stages of grief

Initial shock
Common emotions and experiences—Numbness, disbelief, relief
Task—Accept the reality of the loss

Pangs of grief
Common emotions and experiences—Sadness, anger, guilt, feelings of vulnerability and anxiety, regret, insomnia, social withdrawal, transient auditory and visual hallucinations of the dead person, restlessness, searching behaviour
Task—Experience the pain of grief

Despair
Common emotions and experiences—Loss of meaning and direction in life
Task—Adjust to an environment in which the deceased is missing

Adjustment
Common emotions and experiences—Develop new relationships or interests
Task—Emotionally relocate the deceased to an important but not central place in bereaved person's life and move on

---

Risk factors for poor outcome of bereavement

Predisposing factors
- Ambivalent or dependent relationship
- Multiple prior bereavements
- Previous mental illness, especially depression
- Low self esteem of bereaved person

Around the time of death
- Sudden and unexpected death
- Untimely death of young person
- Preparation for the death
- Stigmatised deaths—Such as AIDS, suicide
- Culpable deaths
- Sex of bereaved person—Elderly male widower
- Caring for deceased person for over 6 months
- Inability to carry out valued religious rituals

After the death
- Level of perceived social support
- Lack of opportunities for new interests
- Stress from other life crises

Generally, sudden and unexpected death is linked with long lasting and high levels of distress, especially if it is associated with violence, suicide, or substance misuse. Cardiovascular disease is the most common cause of sudden death, but in this case a modifying factor may be the timeliness of the death. The sudden death of an elderly person who has lived a full life is generally more acceptable than the death of a young person in a road traffic accident.

In palliative care few deaths are sudden or unexpected to professionals, but it is important to remember that bereaved friends and relatives may have a different view. For informal carers, the strain of caring for a terminally ill person for longer than six months is associated with an increased risk of poor outcome.

People from minority cultural or ethnic groups may experience problems if, at the time of a death, they are not able to follow the rituals and customs they think appropriate.

Deaths carrying a stigma, such as deaths from AIDS or suicide, or deaths for which the bereaved carries some responsibility also bring a higher risk of poor outcome.

After the death, bereaved people who perceive their social support as inadequate are more at risk. Opportunities for developing new interests and relationships may not be available to elderly bereaved people, who may be experiencing reduced mobility or sensory losses because of their own state of health. On the other hand, elderly people may have a more accepting attitude to death because of their experience, while younger people, with higher expectations of the possibility of cure, struggle with its inevitability.

Assessing complicated grief

Since grief and its expression are so much influenced by the society in which a bereaved person lives, and by attitudes and expectations in the immediate family, assessing whether grief is pathological or abnormal is complex. It must take into account several elements.

Intensity and duration of feelings and behaviour—A widow who cries every day about the death of her husband in the first few weeks after his death is within the normal range: if she is doing so 12 months later there is cause for concern. Intense pining, self reproach, and anger are danger signs, as is prolonged withdrawal from social contact. Failure to show any signs of grief is also an indicator, but some people do recover in a few days, especially if they are well prepared for the death.

Culturally determined mourning practices—A mother who maintains the room of her 11 year old son, who died four years ago, as a shrine would be unusual in Britain, but a widow in Japan might talk to her dead husband for the rest of her life as she makes offerings at the household shrine.

Any risk factors likely to make bereavement longer lasting or more deeply challenging.

Bereaved person's personality—Does the person normally express emotion dramatically or is he or she normally self contained and private?

Vulnerable groups

Children

Well meaning adults often wish to protect children from painful events and information during a death in the family but, by doing so, may make children feel the pain of being excluded from events that are very important to them. Children begin to develop an understanding of some aspects of death and bereavement as early as 2 or 3 years. By the age of 5, over half of children have full understanding, and virtually all children will by the age of 8. How early a child develops such

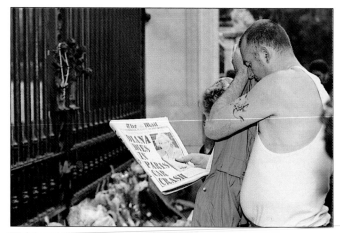

Shock and disbelief are more intense after an unexpected and ultimely death of a young person

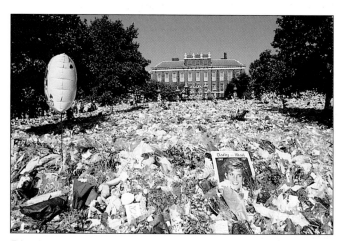

Rituals and public solemnisation of grief are important

How to help in complicated grief

Avoided or repressed grief—Guided mourning that encourages the approach to avoided cues in relation to the dead person

Inability to detach from the dead person, often linked to excessive guilt or self reproach—Saying 'goodbye' to the dead person through writing a letter or having an imaginary conversation with the person supported by a therapist

Chronic grief or avoidance of a new lifestyle—Setting small but progressive goals for change in the context of a therapeutic relationship

Grief after traumatic unexpected death—Consider treatment for post-traumatic stress disorder before treatment for grief reaction

---

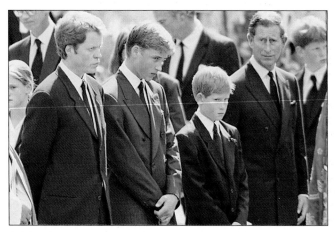

Adults often try to protect children from painful events, including attendance at funerals

understanding depends primarily on whether adults have given truthful and sensitive explanations of any experience of death that the child may have had, and only secondarily on the level of cognitive development.

When a death is about to occur or has occurred, it is important to discuss with parents what experience of death their children have and what they have been told about the current situation, and to encourage the children to ask any questions. Parents are the best people to talk to their children, but they may need support and advice from professionals. Storybooks and workbooks on death and bereavement have been produced for children.

Parents may be preoccupied with the practical difficulties of caring for someone who is dying or overwhelmed with their own grief. In this case it may be useful to involve concerned family friends or teachers. For adolescents struggling to develop their individuality and independence, their peer group may be a helpful resource, particularly if it includes someone who has also experienced the death of a family member.

Confused elderly people and those with learning disabilities

The needs of these groups for help in dealing with bereavement have often been ignored. Repeated explanations and supported involvement in important events, such as the funeral and visiting the grave, have been shown to reduce the repetitious questions about the whereabouts of the dead person by confused elderly people or difficult and withdrawn behaviour in people with learning disabilities. This makes their continuing care less demanding for both family and professional carers.

What helps?

Identifying people potentially at risk in bereavement—Much pathology can be avoided by work before the death to minimise the effect of factors that increase risk of poor outcome.

Being present at the death, seeing the body afterwards, and attending the funeral or memorial service—These are helpful provided the bereaved person (including children) wishes to participate and is prepared for these events.

Providing information to bereaved people about the feelings they may have and about sources of voluntary support through leaflets or empathetic personal contact.

Counselling targeted at those in high risk categories, particularly those who perceive their social supports to be unhelpful. Counselling to unselected groups shows little benefit. Visits by trained bereavement volunteers have been shown to reduce use of general practitioners' services.

Opportunities to meet in bereavement groups, where people can safely test out the often disturbing feelings, questions, and thoughts that they have with others going through similar experiences.

There is no single intervention that meets the needs of all bereaved people, but there is an increasing range of resources for them to draw on. Most hospices offer a bereavement service to families with whom they are in contact. This may range from a telephone call or individual visits by volunteers to group meetings. Many areas have branches of the national self help organisations. In addition psychologists, community psychiatric nurses, and social workers with an interest in health care have the skills to work with bereaved people whose problems require more than the loving support of family and friends or the sharing of experiences with other bereaved people.

Books for children to read or use

Couldrick A. *When your mum or dad has cancer*. Oxford: Sobell Publications, 1991

Heegard M. *When someone has a serious illness*. Minneapolis: Woodland Press, 1991 (workbook)

Heegard M. *When someone very special dies*. Minneapolis: Woodland Press, 1988 (workbook)

Mellonie B, Ingpen R. *Lifetimes*. Melbourne: Dragon's World, 1983

Stickney D. *Water bugs and dragonflies*. London: Mowbray, 1982

Varley S. *Badger's parting gifts*. London: Picture Lions, 1982

Williams G, Ross J. *When people die*. Midlothian: Macdonald Publishers, 1983 (for teenagers)

Organisations for bereaved people

Compassionate Friends
- 53 North Street, Bristol BS53 1EN (tel 0117 966 5202)
- National organisation with local branches. Offers befriending to bereaved parents after loss of child of any age

Cruse Bereavement Care
- Cruse House, 126 Sheen Road, Richmond TW9 1UR (tel 0181 332 7227)
- National organisation with local branches. Offers counselling and befriending, home visits, and social meetings. Some specialist services

Jewish Bereavement Counselling Service
- PO Box 6748, London N3 3BX (tel 0181 349 0839)
- Counselling by trained volunteers. Telephone helpline

Lesbian and Gay Bereavement Project
- AIDS Education Unit, Vaughan M Williams Centre, Colindale Hospital, London NW9 5HG (tel 0181 200 0511)
- Advice, support, and counselling for bereaved gay men, lesbians, and their families and friends. Education. Telephone helpline (evenings)

National Association of Bereavement Services
- 20 Norton Folgate, London E1 6DB (tel 0171 247 0617)
- Referral agency. Publishes directory of bereavement and loss services. Support organisation for bereavement services

SANDS (Stillbirth and Neonatal Death Society)
- 28 Portland Place, London W1N 4DE (tel 0171 436 5881)
- Support for parents after stillbirth or neonatal death

The painting by Fourie is reproduced with permission of Bridgeman Art Library and the pictures of mourning after the death of Diana, Princess of Wales, are reproduced with permission of Rex Features. Frances Sheldon is Macmillan lecturer in psychosocial palliative care at the University of Southampton.

Index

Index